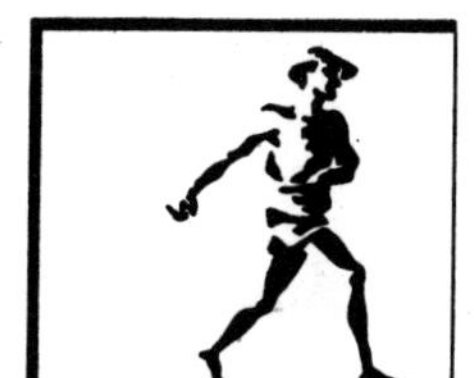

SIMON AND SCHUSTER
N E W Y O R K

Kathryn Klinger's First Book of Beauty

Photographs by Harry Langdon

Published by Simon and Schuster
A Division of Simon & Schuster, Inc.
Simon & Schuster Building
Rockefeller Center
1230 Avenue of the Americas
New York, New York 10020
SIMON AND SCHUSTER and colophon are registered trademarks of Simon & Schuster, Inc.
Designed by Karolina Harris

Manufactured in the United States of America
10 9 8 7 6 5 4 3 2 1

Library of Congress Cataloging in Publication Data
Klinger, Kathryn.
Kathryn Klinger's First book of beauty.
1. Beauty, Personal. I. Title.
RA778.K7223 1984 646.7'2 83-20411
ISBN 0-671-46283-0

All exercise photos by Harry Langdon except for those on pages 53, 54, and 135, which are by Robert Berger.
Illustrations by Glenn Tunstull.

Acknowledgments

Special thanks to Suzy Kalter, my friend and partner who helped me to write this book; to all the loyal employees of Georgette Klinger, Inc., who have watched me grow up and who continue to give their best to us; to Wayne Webb, a longtime friend; to Mike Dougherty and Harriet Sacks for their support and caring.

Thanks to Patricia Soliman, my hardworking and wonderful editor; to Harry Langdon and his team of magicians, who made the photography go so smoothly; William Martinez who did my hair; Glenn Tunstull, who drew the illustrations. Thanks also to Dr. Debra C. Kalter, who read the text to make sure it was medically accurate; to Dr. Richard Leiber, who checked the dental chapter; and to Dr. William Fein, who made sure the eye chapter is outta sight.

ACKNOWLEDGMENTS

To my wonderful mother, Georgette Klinger,
without whom there would be no book!
And in memory of my father.
And to my practically perfect husband, Rudy Belton,
with love for his constant support and understanding.

Contents

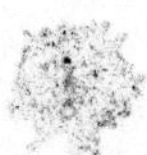

CONTENTS

Five: Teeth and Mouth 83

Six: Eyes 96

CONTENTS

Seven: Hands and Feet 110

Eight: Makeup 124

Nine: Plastic Surgery 152

Ten: Health and Exercise 163

Preface

True Confessions

To me, I was a mess.

I had hoped to have been born beautiful and to continue that way for the rest of my life, but it didn't work.

Oh, I guess I was born beautiful enough—I was healthy, I had the requisite number of fingers and toes, and while I didn't have hair, I did keep my blue eyes. To my parents, I was always beautiful.

But I knew better. Once I was old enough to discover that my mother was not only a natural beauty, but one of the world's foremost experts on beauty, health and skin care, I considered skipping right back into the nursery and locking the door.

As the "daughter of," I always felt that I couldn't have any flaws. I assumed people were looking twice as hard at me, trying to measure me in my mother's image. I scrutinized myself far more closely than any other girl need ever do. What I saw in the mirror was deeply distressing!

I had oily skin.

I had a pimple on my face.

I had fine, limp hair.

My nose did not turn up in pert defiance of gravity the way my friend Lillian's did.

If my mother hadn't taught me a few tricks of the trade, if I hadn't gone to cosmetology school, if I had been unable to find my own identity and my own look, I surely would have perished from self-doubt. Luckily for me, before I could develop a terminal inferiority complex, I was able to learn that very few people are born beautiful. But anyone can—and should—develop her own style and then do her best to look as beautiful as she can.

I've taught myself how to maximize my good points and minimize my flaws. I've also learned not to be obsessed with my looks, to take good care of my skin and appearance and to concentrate on other qualities—to do what I can to make myself look good and then get on with the rest of my life. And every young woman can do what I did.

Growing up in the beauty business (I began by putting stamps on mail-order packages when I was six, coming in after school, and worked my way up to telephone answering at age twelve), I have educated my eyes to perceive the myriad possibilities for making what God gave you look just a little bit better. (Okay, a lot better.) I spent most of my school years, and almost all my travel time, looking at people's faces, wondering what could be done to improve their looks. My mother used to embarrass me by occasionally stopping someone on a plane and offering her a helpful makeup trick or skin-care tip. I was never bold enough to do that. But I have to admit that while my teachers were busy grading me on my schoolwork, I was perpetually giving them mental grades on how well they had put themselves together. I was forever dying to change their lipstick color or advise them on how to tweeze their eyebrows properly.

It was a relief to graduate from college (Yes, I flew home on weekends when I needed a facial. Wouldn't you?) and go on to cosmetology school so I could get my training and begin to dole out the advice, information and tips teeming inside me all those years. After all, I'd been working on myself since I was twelve. I still wish I had a smaller nose, longer lashes and a bit more bosom, but I've learned to do the best with what I have. And more important, I've seen myself blossom, so I know that no matter how gawky you are now, you can look and *feel* gorgeous —if you work at it. I did it, and a lot of other people I know have done it. Now it's your turn.

Kathryn Klinger's First Book of Beauty

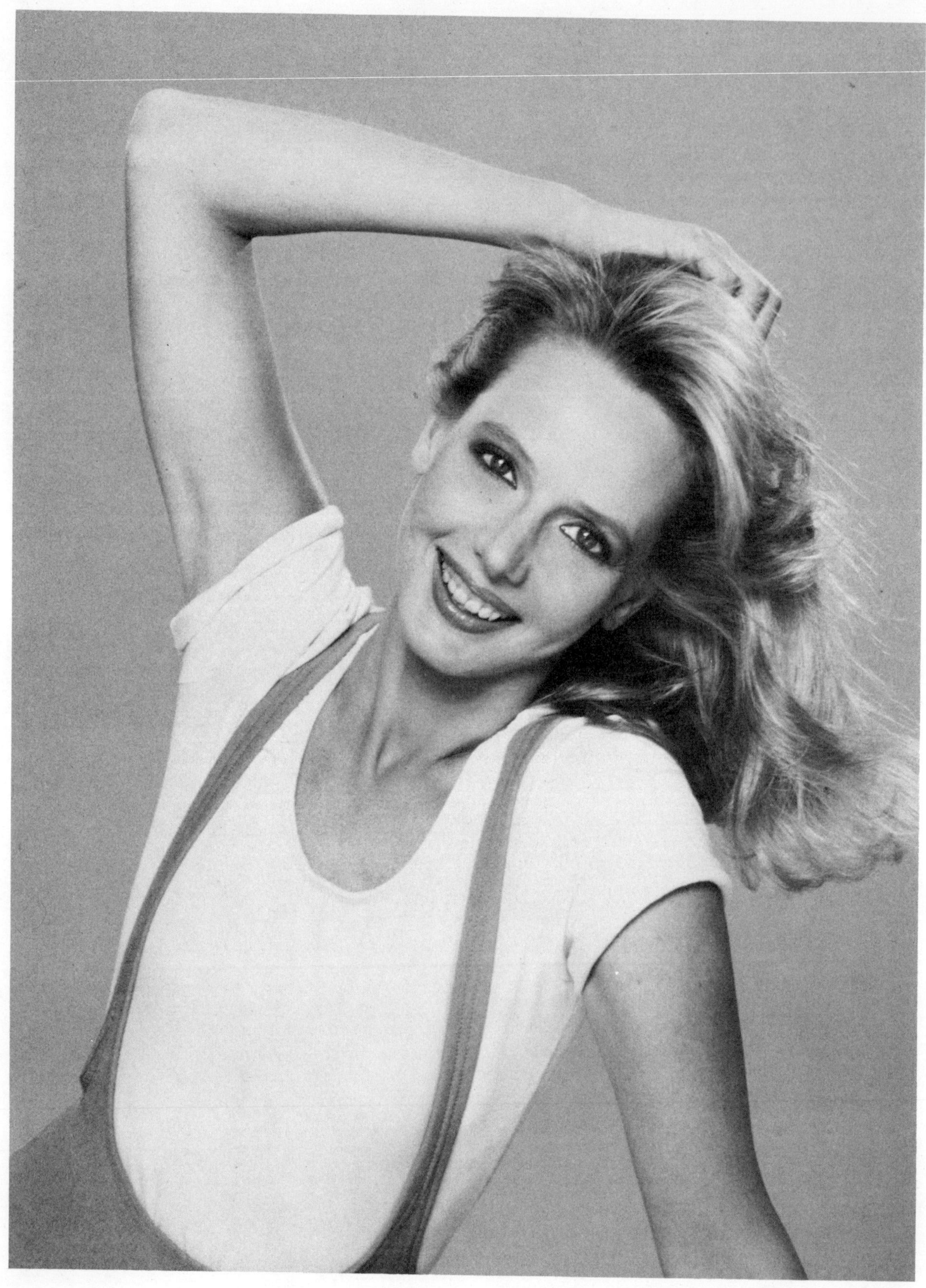

One

Beauty Habits

Look in the mirror and what do you see? The beginnings of a beautiful woman. Maybe you don't think so, but I'm the expert—not you. Beauty is largely a matter of good habits. The things you do to your face and body now will be with you until the day you die. How attractive you become—and stay; how you age; whether you walk into a room with the bounce and shine of a winner or slouch toward obscurity are all alternatives that depend on you and your attention to detail. You can go a long way in life—probably into your mid-thirties or early forties—without caring for yourself. The dividends may loom so far ahead you can't imagine yourself twenty years from now. But somewhere along the line when you look in the mirror you will know either triumph or despair. The choice is yours. If you spend an hour a day taking care of your good looks, you'll always have something to be proud of. If you don't build good beauty habits now, you will never be able to buy back lost time. The looks you crave don't come out of a jar. They come from the heart—and the head. Be smart now, and you'll never be sorry.

BEAUTY FACTS

To me, there are two basic facts:

■ There is no excuse for not looking your most beautiful.

■ Every woman is different and is therefore beautiful in a different way.

Women who try to look like other women will inevitably be frustrated all their lives. There will always be richer and more beautiful women. You can't compete with all of them, so you might as well compete with yourself. Women who have a strong sense of self can develop a look that makes them feel in control—feel the power that comes only from self-confidence. The power of a beautiful person.

So dump your fairy-tale notions of looking like the princess in the storybook your mother used to read you. Forget about the girl you saw in the Calvin Klein jeans ad just the other day. Pay no heed to the razzle-dazzle of the Girl from Ipanema. Simply find the place within that makes you feel good about yourself, and go for it on a daily basis. Don't measure yourself by your mother or your sister or your best friend.

This is the real importance of being earnest: *being you.*

Get into the habit of looking your best. Learn your body. Get to know how often your hair has to be washed. Don't go by what some expert said on a TV show. Go by what's right for *your* hair. Know how long your manicure lasts, when your skin breaks out, why and how best to care for those bumps and blotches. The more you learn and the more you practice, the more you will do for yourself and your future.

A woman goes through many stages as she progresses from child to adult. After the awkward years, she begins to create her own style. Often the girls who start life "pretty" are slow to develop personal style because they get by on being a pretty face. Less attractive girls know they have to work on their looks, to achieve their own panache. They become the women we envy because they're so pulled-together, so classy and so stylish.

I don't care if your nose is crooked, your teeth are uneven and your skin deeply troubled—you can conquer these problems. You just need the knowledge and the commitment. The idea that beauty comes from "within" is nonsense. Yes, health and happiness are reflected in how you look—true enough. But *real* beauty comes from intelligence, education and skill. There's waking up beautiful and there's walking out the door beautiful; and I assure you, very few women in the world wake up beautiful. But every woman can walk out the door beautiful.

Maybe you'll never be a classic beauty. Maybe your face will never grace the cover of a glossy magazine. But you can have a special kind of beauty nonetheless. You can find the kind of beauty that is yours—yours alone—and you can build it into the quiet confidence that doesn't have to shout; that simply whispers, "I am special."

Beauty is not only in the eye of the beholder. It's also in the soul of the owner. It comes with the determination to be beautiful, and the discipline to follow up your determination. When you've put all the necessary time and effort into your looks, you're proud of the results. You have the confidence to go on to the more important things in life, feeling that you can conquer the world. You get that confidence not from giving yourself a pep talk, but from knowing that you've done the best you can in taking care of yourself. Beauty may not be the most important thing in life, but it is an international passport to the best. Have you ever noticed that the attractive people get the choice tables in restaurants, the fastest service in department stores, the small favors from strangers? It's no coincidence. Whether you like it or not, appearance counts. When you decide to be the best person you can be, you are admitting that the world cares if your hair is clean, if your breath is sweet and your skin radiantly glowing.

Looking your best is not a matter so much of being lucky as it is of being smart—smart enough to find your look and learn how to maintain it. Once you learn to take care of what you have, to use your good points—and your bad ones too—to your personal advantage, you will turn into your very own magician. It takes a *mature* person to be able to assess herself objectively—to accept the facts, change what can be changed and learn to live with the rest. And that is the secret of *real* beauty!

Beauty is not simply a matter of having wheat-blond hair or sky-blue eyes or a turned-up nose. The national model seems to be the cover girl—Brooke Shields, Farrah Fawcett or Christie Brinkley. All over the country, women aged five to fifty try to look like these paragons rather than be themselves! In Europe, on the other hand, it is not unusual to see a model on the cover of a fashion magazine whose nose is crooked or bumpy or who has a mole on her cheek. Perfectionism is an American mania that is invading the realm of individual beauty. In trying to look perfect, women forfeit their individual beauty. They become obsessed with looking like someone else; they want a nose of "perfect" length and shape, hair styled in the manner of the latest beauty superstar. They want all the character taken out of their faces and a doll-like perfection painted on instead. They are afraid to be true to themselves for fear of not fitting in.

Farrah Fawcett has her own style—she *made* her look. But when millions of women decided to do their hair just like Farrah's, they surrendered their own natural appeal. The copies are never as beautiful as the original. (They may be *striking*, but never beautiful.) Sophia Loren has created a look for herself, even though her nose is large and her features are not classically perfect. Yet Sophia has an original beauty that no woman can copy. That's beauty! That's style!

Trying to conform to someone else's notion of beauty also makes you supremely self-conscious. You can't be comfortable while you are trying to look like someone else; you will be at ease when you develop your own style and let your own beauty shine through. So tear down your Farrah poster, toss out your magazine covers. Let's get to the truth about you. Let's work on making *you* the star.

CHECK OUT YOUR ASSETS

Before we begin improving you, take a look at what heredity and chance have given you:

■ "I've got thunder thighs, just like my mom. There's nothing I can do about them."

■ "My mother and sister had problem skin. It cleared up when they went to college. So I guess it's just a matter of waiting."

■ "My nose is a bit of a beak, but it's my family trademark."

Before you go too far in analyzing your looks, take a look at your family tree and check out your assets—and your debits. Use your knowledge of genetics to help your cause. Not as an excuse. Take pride in the good things that have been passed your way. Spot trouble zones before they become a problem for you.

Sum up your mother's looks. Chances are, you will age in much the same way—in terms of both your face and your figure. Is Mom looking a little old before her time? Has she spent too many hours in the sun? Is her hair beginning to gray? Or are you considering applying for a job in one of those commercials where you can't tell the mother from the daughter?

Heredity shows up sooner or later. This is often a difficult concept for people under thirty. When you are a teenager or in your early twenties, it's very hard to look at yourself as you are and imagine what you will look like in another twenty or thirty years. If you see a family resemblance between yourself and your mother, it's important to realize that you can control some of the beauty aspects of your own aging process. The choices you make today *will* matter later. The pimple you squeeze today may scar you forever. If you don't like your mother's lined face, have you stopped your own sunbathing?

If good skin runs in your family, congratulations. The chances are excellent you will have easy-to-care-for skin for a lifetime. That doesn't mean you don't have to look after it, or that sun won't parch your face or wind wrinkle your brow. Good skin endures when you take care of it.

If good skin is not a family characteristic, you can still achieve it. In fact, even if you come from a family plagued by bad skin, you are not necessarily condemned to the same fate. With professional help you can change the way your skin behaves, even if you can't tinker with your genetic code.

Your skeleton is yours to keep, and so are your genes; but beyond that, you can alter just about anything you want. It may not be worth it to you to turn your baby-blue eyes green with a pair of contact lenses (especially if you don't even need glasses!), but you can keep your figure from spreading, your skin from breaking out and those crow's-feet from dancing across your face for just a little bit longer.

Go through some family photo albums and chart your beauty history. History repeats itself, you know, so get a good idea now of what the future may hold in store.

FAMILY HISTORY

As you riffle through the album pages, from generation to generation, respond True or False to these statements:

1. My mother has always looked older than her age.
2. You can see the family resemblance between my mother and her sisters.
3. The men on both sides of my family seem to age better than the women.
4. Good skin seems to run in my family.
5. Many members of my family had acne.
6. Acne affected them during their teen years only.
7. Acne affected them throughout their lives.
8. After about age 35, my mother began to look middle-aged.
9. My mother has had wrinkles and lines since she was 35–40.

10. Other members of her family have the exact same type of skin.
11. Skin is bad only on the members of my family who were active in outdoor sports or were sun worshipers.
12. Sensitive skin runs in my family; rashes and allergies are not uncommon.
13. I have the same body type as other members of my family.
14. Other members of my family have always had to watch their weight.
    a. flabby thighs? b. sagging seat? c. potbelly? d. wide buttocks?
15. Other members of my family are overweight or obese.
16. Poor eyesight is a family trait.
17. Other members of my family have needed orthodontia.

To Rate Your Own Possibilities

For each statement to which you have responded True, a likelihood exists that you too have a predisposition toward this tendency. You inherit only a tendency, not a condition. So what you do *will* affect your looks. Wrinkles and premature aging can be prevented with proper skin care and the use of sunblocks. If there is a predilection toward acne, but your skin is still clear, check with your family doctor or cosmetologist about preventive diets and skin-care treatments. If other members of your family have had a weight problem, prevent your own hips from spreading with a diligent exercise program and a sensible diet. Body type is hereditary, but weight problems *can* be controlled or prevented. You have the power to control much of your beauty future.

LEGACIES

Genes aren't the only things that are passed on in families. Each has its own legacy of stories, anecdotes, old wives' tales and half-truths; there is a family grapevine and a sisterhood of small talk that weaves its way through generations. Sometimes family beauty tips turn out to be helpful. Many times—unfortunately—the information is hearsay or myth.

How many of these statements do you think are true? (Circle Fact or Fiction.)

- Only soap and water can really clean your skin.
  Fact *Fiction*
- You must brush your hair 100 strokes to make it really shine.
  Fact *Fiction*
- You must not wash your hair when you have your period.
  Fact *Fiction*

- The sun will clear up acne.
  Fact *Fiction*
- Most mouthwashes kill germs and fight bad breath and tooth decay.
  Fact *Fiction*
- If you pull out a gray hair, six new ones will grow in its place.
  Fact *Fiction*
- Sex will clear up acne.
  Fact *Fiction*

Okay, let's see how you did. This quiz is easy to score because all these statements are old wives' tales. Some are half-truths, some are based on misinformation and some are just plain false. Add to these the little tips your own family has been passing on to you, like the right way to tweeze your eyebrows or to put on makeup or wash your hair, and you could be defeating your own beauty program by accident! Never take a beauty tip for granted. Question information and test it yourself; then make up your own mind.

Unless your mother is an expert on skin care (as mine is) or your sister has a cosmetician's license, I think you should investigate family how-tos and compare them with experts' opinions. Friends and relatives mean well, but they may be giving you fuzzy facts. Be wary.

When I was in high school, my best friend was named Nancy. Nancy had olive skin, blue-black hair and coal-black eyes beneath her bushy black brows. I had pale blond hair, no discernible eyebrows, water-blue eyes and ghost-white skin. Yet Nancy and I spent all our after-school hours together, one of us rooted in front of the bathroom sink, the other perched on the toilet with a hand mirror, both dedicated to helping each other toward "beauty." We used the same foundation, the same rouge and the same green eye shadow, blind to the fact that we had entirely different coloring and therefore entirely different beauty needs. All we did was give each other misinformation and reinforce bad habits.

So do me a favor, and go to an expert for the facts. If you want to get involved in some harmless experimenting with family or friends, go ahead. But if you want to look better right away, don't waste your time. Go to a pro instead.

WHEN TO BEGIN YOUR BEAUTY PLAN

Of course, it's never too soon to set up a program for sensible skin care—the earlier the better. But you will know when it's time to seek out some expert advice when you take my Telltale Nose Test, below. When you pass, make an appointment with a specialist and begin to talk seriously about your face and figure.

Even if you don't pass my nose test yet, chances are that if you're approaching puberty, your body is beginning to change and the peer pressure to know a little bit more about glamour is beginning to intensify—if your interest in the opposite sex is growing—it's time to see a professional.

KATHRYN KLINGER'S TELLTALE NOSE TEST

This is one test on which failure carries no penalty. To me, "failing" the test simply means you are not yet ready for professional advice. "Passing" means it's time to see a cosmetologist. Take a long, careful look at your nose, especially at the curved part where the nostrils join the cheeks and lead to the bridge. If you see clogged pores or blackheads (seen as black dots), you have identified the enemy and "passed" the nose test. It's time for professional guidance. If your skin is still baby-perfect, you have "failed" the need for expert help; but keep checking every month or so.

Once you go to see someone about your skin (the oilier your skin, by the way, the earlier in your life it will be), it's time to set up your own beauty regimen of good habits.

You're going to have to learn to:

- ignore the advertising and media pressure that will try to influence you toward the Big Sell;
- do things differently because of age, environment or changing hormones;
- not rely exclusively on handed-down helpful hints.

Blackheads and clogged pores

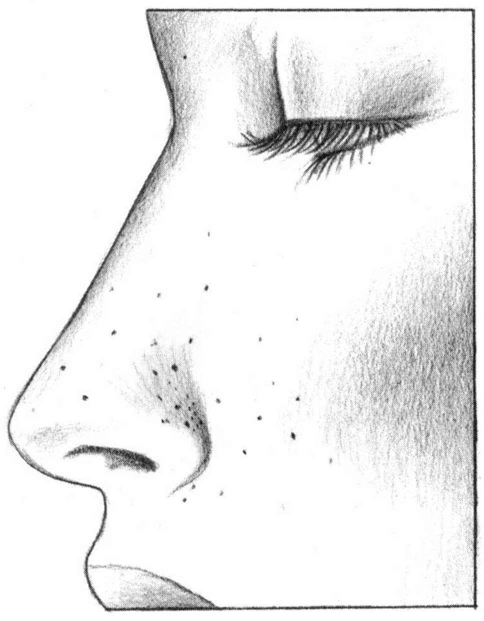

Clear, healthy skin

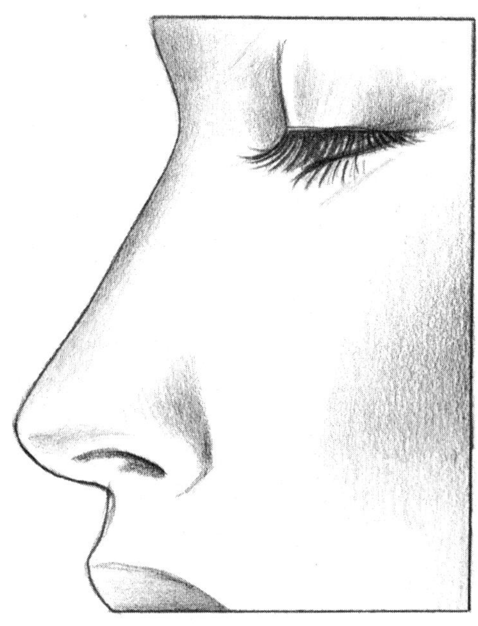

GETTING SMART

If you don't seek the professional help you need, one of three things has happened to you:

- You're confused by all the ads you see in magazines and on TV;
- You've gotten lazy;
- You've developed a defeatist attitude and have given up.

When you're young it's particularly easy to postpone things that don't seem important. If you are confused about an issue, you hope that by ignoring it, you may wake up one day and find the problem has solved itself. But beauty care doesn't work that way, so it's important you get smart at an early age. Work through your confusion now.

- *Confused?* Do all those ads, all that packaging make your head spin? Think about beauty advertising for a minute. Its sole purpose is to make each person feel insecure enough to go out and buy yet another product. Models are booked on the basis of their beauty; ads are created to make the reader feel *less beautiful* than the model. The illusion is that if you use the product, you will look like the model. In reality, the model selling the acne lotion may never have have had a pimple in her life and certainly wouldn't have gotten the assignment if she had had one that day. The woman selling the wrinkle cream is ten years too young to even worry about wrinkles!

Most of us never see the elaborate preparation that goes on during a photo session. The gorgeous photogenic face that stares up at you from the pages of your favorite magazine gets a lot of help. At the photography session there are a hairdresser to make sure not one little hair is out of place, a fashion consultant to see that every fold of the dress lies properly and, of course, a makeup artist to create the face that many women will try to imitate after they purchase the product advertised. Hundreds of pictures later, one photo will be chosen, retouched and sent to print. Retouching is a kind of magic; a blemish can be made to disappear completely, wrinkles can be softened and made indiscernible, even an expression can be altered. Hundreds of hours of time and energy will have been invested to garner this one picture.

Analyze what you read. Ask yourself, "What is the ad really saying?" Many ads are beautifully worded, but filled with empty promises. Learn to look at an ad and say to yourself, "Wow, that model looks beautiful, but she probably doesn't wake up that way." That's the Big Sell—identify it as such, and don't let it confuse you.

- *Lazy?* Too much homework? Too many errands? Just don't want to take the time out for your face and figure? When you're young, it's sometimes hard to understand exactly what you are working toward and that today's habits really *do* matter. It's easier to go soft; to try to postpone the facts for a while; to ignore those bumps on your nose, to pretend they'll go away. Ignoring is the beginning of a bad habit; being lazy about your looks is almost like a virus.

You start off by ignoring the little signs that whisper, "Help me! Help me!" Then the whisper turns to a shout as one area after another calls for more than first aid. Skin problems develop, your thighs ripple a little more than they should (especially at your age!), a birthmark that should have been removed years ago mars your otherwise attractive complexion. Sometime between your twenty-fifth and thirty-fifth birthdays, tomorrow has caught up with you. While that date may seem light-years distant right now, it'll be a shame to have thrown away your looks—to look forty-five just as you turn thirty-five—all because you were too passive and didn't get off on the right foot when you were growing up.

Even if you are happily married, you cannot ignore the needs of your beauty program. You don't have to go to bed with curlers in your hair and a pound of cream on your cheeks; but if you don't keep up with the basics, one day you'll find yourself looking older than your friends, worrying if your husband thinks you're fading, or even divorced or widowed and wanting to look your best as you set out on an adventurous new chapter in your life. Sorry, Women's Lib, but men *do* count! It's false confidence to think you will never age or will not have a need to be attractive in the years to come. Remember, lazy today means sorry tomorrow, and being smart means taking care of yourself every single day.

■ *Defeated?* You think there's no hope? So many young women look in their mirrors and cry themselves to sleep. Many have serious skin problems; others just aren't satisfied with what they see. Instead of taking a positive attitude and deciding to get help, they give up. No matter how bad your skin (Believe me, I've seen plenty of cases of acne) or how low your own estimation of your looks, there is always something that can be done to make you look and feel better. You don't deserve to punish yourself by suffering. Go after results and you'll get them!

COMMITMENT MEANS DISCIPLINE

If you really are going to take your future into your own hands, you're going to have to be committed to me and to yourself. You can't do good works only occasionally and expect to reap the benefits. You can't be lazy *some* of the time. You can't expect to keep your skin clear and your hair shimmering if you don't follow through on the proper methods. Each body will have its own requirements. But the person who is a winner will work to discover those requirements and to meet them energetically until she looks as good as she can.

If you want to make changes, you've come to the right place. I can tell you a lot about what's needed. But I can't do the work for you. Only you can do that. And once changes are made, only you can maintain your enhanced beauty. Beauty is a lifelong commitment. There are no miracles; no easy formulas. And you'll gain nothing from this book unless you're serious about making that commitment.

Take a good look at the older women you know. Some look dramatically better than others. It is obvious which ones have a lifelong dedication to beauty. Some may have worked a little harder than others, but they'll all tell you the results are definitely worth it.

Two

Healthy Skin

Your own skin-care routine plays a crucial role in how your face reacts to wear and tear. Girls who begin proper skin-care techniques when they are pre-teens have fewer problems over the span of their lives than those who take their good skin for granted until they are thirty-five, then shrug and decide they'll get a face lift in ten years. Surprisingly, a bad skin can actually be an ultimate advantage. Girls with problem skin grow into women with healthy skin-care habits. The girl with the good skin early on is not always inspired to establish vital routines and, in the long run, may have a higher price to pay.

A lot of the problems skin encounters can be controlled by you. You just need to know how and to care enough to give your skin the very best.

If you squint or frown or have any other habitual facial expressions that cause lines when you speak or listen, work on breaking the habit. Ask a good friend if you are uncertain about having any such expressions. Often we don't realize we are raising our brows when we're surprised or interested, at the same time causing an unnecessary line. What you can do is 1) become aware and 2) massage against the line or potential line with your fingertips—almost like ironing it out.

Now let's talk about the Good Sister and the Bad Sister. Not the proverbial Good Girls and Bad Girls Mother has been lecturing you about, but the Skin Sisters. Both were born with the same skin type and the same genetic heritage of fairly good skin.

One sister was a picky eater—she didn't like vegetables at all and hardly ever ate salad. She was a "meat and potatoes" girl, but also enjoyed frequent hamburgers and pizza. Since she didn't have a weight problem, she would usually hit the refrigerator for a soft drink when she came home from school before doing her homework. She liked to read a lot and didn't go in for sports. She was careful to be neat and clean, of course, but she had no established beauty program. She washed her hair, she slept in rollers, she had a perm when everyone else did, she wore the latest styles, she used the same amount of makeup that all the girls in her class did and she was popular enough. She didn't have

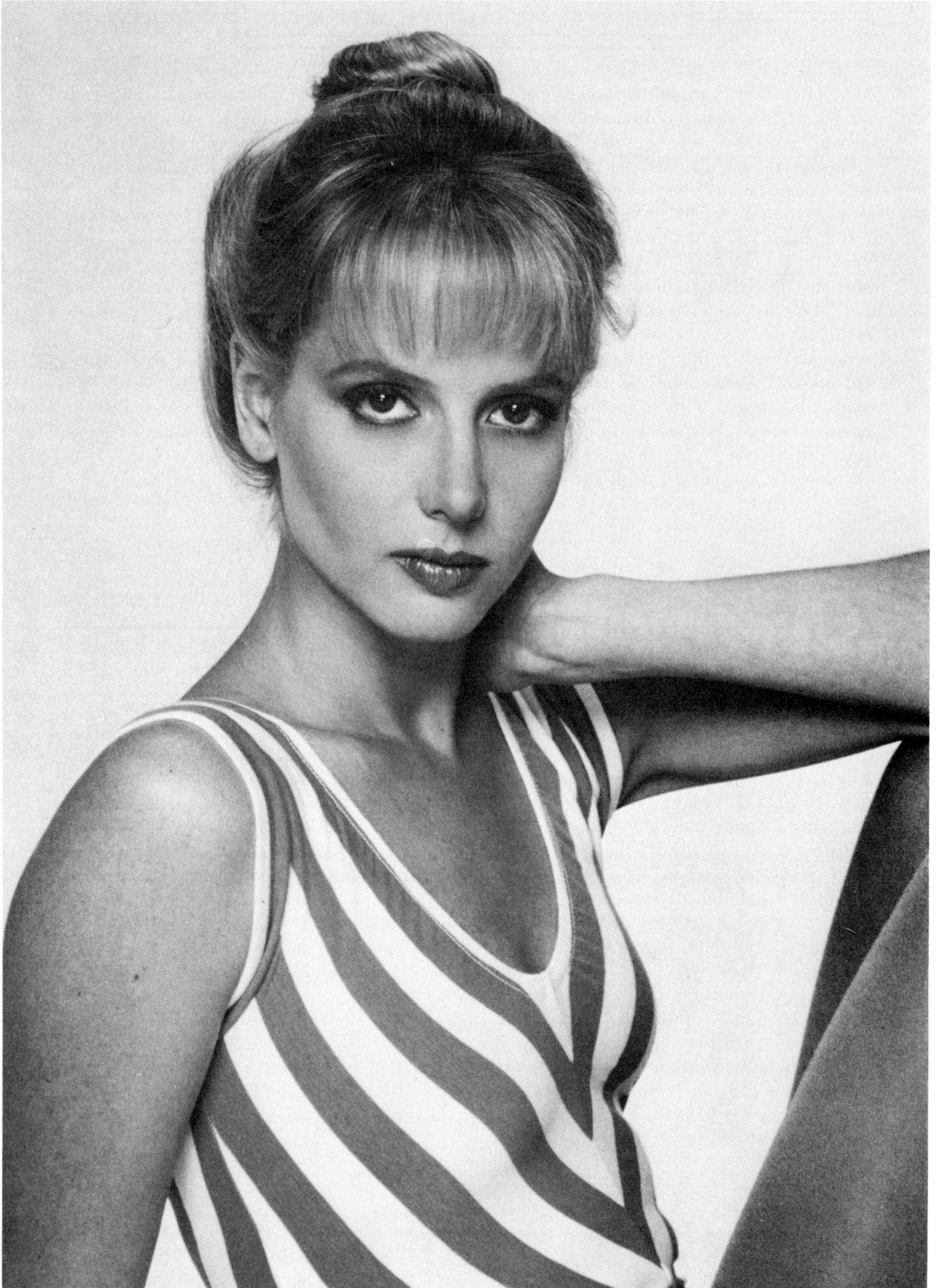

many pimples, except sometimes right before her period, when she would simply bake in the sun to dry them out. She wasn't too careful about taking off her makeup, because some nights she was "just too beat." And she grew up to be a very fine woman.

Her sister had a different lifestyle even when they were kids. She always watched what she ate and made an effort to eat green and yellow vegetables, because she knew they were good for her. She avoided soft drinks, never got involved in drinking or drugs and had pizza or burgers only as an occasional treat. She jogged with her parents every morning before school and had a fifteen-minute morning and night beauty routine that she practiced even on weekends and holidays and at summer camp. She didn't care for lying in the sun, and always used a sunscreen when exercising outdoors; she used both moisturizer and eye cream regularly. And she grew up to be a very fine woman.

For most of their years, the sisters did not look remarkably different. The one who ignored her skin had no major problems; the one who took care of herself had no halo hovering over her head. Only an expert could have told the difference.

When one sister was thirty-two, the other was thirty-five. The Bad Sister, who was actually the younger, looked ten years older than the Good Sister. And it was too late to make much difference to her skin's future. The damage had been silently and secretly done over the years. And once done, it is irreversible.

BUILDING GOOD SKIN

Your skin is your body's largest organ, and it is a faithful indicator of your health. People who "look sick" usually have sallow skin. Likewise, people who don't feed their bodies right can count on seeing rashes, breakouts, flakiness and color variances.

People who don't remove their makeup at night, who have bad personal habits, who lack the foresight to look ahead ten or twenty years and who thoughtlessly play skin doctor to themselves all build poor foundations for their skin's future.

Since my mother was a specialist, I had to grow up listening to unsolicited advice—advice I couldn't believe was true because it was so directly contrary to what all my friends were hearing from *their* moms. We used to summer at Lake Placid, and Mother's first rule was DON'T GO OUT IN THE SUN!

How I hated that advice. Every girl I *knew* went sunbathing and obsessively cultivated her tan. Some mothers bought their daughters the latest tanning lotions, or helped them mix baby oil and iodine with cocoa butter. *My* mother came running after me with a sunblock and tried to shelter me in the shade. Now, of course, I wish I'd listened to her and hadn't wanted a tan so badly. But back then, twenty-five years ago, nobody else's mother told her the sun was bad for her skin.

Then Mother would say: DON'T USE SOAP!

I can't remember ever using soap. On my face, that is. Soap is a very good product, ideal for cleaning the body. But not the face. So while my friends were lathering, I learned to use cleansing lotion on a piece of cotton pulled from a cotton roll (not the kind that comes in a bag of ready-made puffs).

Now, I'm not saying my mother was perfect. After all, there was the time when she finally let me have bangs and cut them for me herself. And cut and cut and cut. Too short? So short we could hardly find them! So let your mother practice only what she knows. If she's a hairstylist, by all means, let her cut your hair. If she runs her own national skin-care salon, don't let her cut your hair, but pay attention to her beauty advice. If she's a mechanic, trust her when it comes to your bicycle.

Mom means best, but there are new scientific developments she may not know about; and beyond that, she may not have the same skin type you do. If you find her advice is working, stick with it. But if you're breaking out or have some questions Mom just can't answer, do both of you a favor and see a specialist.

THE SKIN TYPES

Dry skin: If you have dry skin, your younger years will be blissful, with a minimal amount of breakout. Your skin will probably be clear and smooth. Of course, as you get older you will have problems oily skins don't have, such as premature aging, flakiness and that dry, tight feeling. Your skin may not be as soft or supple as you'd like. Dry skin has a tendency to age faster than other types and over the long run requires more care than oily skin.

Oily skin: Oily skin is never seen as an advantage by teenagers who bemoan the pimples that invariably accompany hormonal changes. But the older you get, the more slowly oily skin ages and the less work it needs to stay glowing. You also save money on creams and lubricants.

Combination skin: Combination skin is sometimes labeled either oily or dry and treated as such—which is a big mistake. It is really like having two separate skins to treat. Take care of each skin accordingly. You will need two cleansers—otherwise neither part will get adequate care. An astringent for oily skin can destroy the delicate drier area, while a moisturizer for dry skin may cause a blemish to break out on the oily area. It's also possible that you are "O" and "D" in the same places; this means that underneath the surface of your skin is oily, but you have dried out the top layer so it looks as though you have dry skin. This usually triggers an unhappy cycle, because you try to combat the dryness with cream and the cream causes the oily skin to break out even more. What you need is a milder cleanser and perhaps a light water-based moisturizer that you use very sparingly two or three times a week.

Normal skin: Neither too oily, too dry nor any combination of them, normal skin has small pores, no flakiness, no oily feel and resembles a child's. The other skin types are not "abnormal," so don't be upset if you don't have "normal" skin. Few people do!

The ideal skin: It should be soft to the touch and look and feel smooth when you run your fingertips over it. It will have a healthy glow, free of open pores, blackheads or bumps. The skin's color will be a healthy rosy shade, not gray or lackluster, and no broken capillaries (red veins) should be visible.

ASSESSING YOUR SKIN

Much of what you will do in your lifetime of skin care depends on what type of skin you have and how to treat it. You'll have to do a little Nancy Drewing on your own to discover exactly what type is yours.

Don't make guesses, don't ask friends. This is something you need to do by yourself:

1. Pull your hair away from your face (use a coated elastic band—or shower cap if you have short hair) and clean your skin as best you can. Wait one hour for your skin to balance out and for your natural oils to reappear.

2. Go outside with a magnifying mirror. If it's not possible to go outside, stand by a window, with the lights off, in a room with neutral-colored walls. (No green walls—you'll look extremely ill.) Avoid neon and artificial light.

3. Look over your face, section by section. Sketch your face on a piece of paper (a big circle will do just fine). As you go through the sections, mark the picture with your findings.

A: *Nose:* is it shiny or matte?

If it's shiny, you have oily skin. Write "O" on your nose in the sketch.

If your nose is matte, you have normal or dry skin. Write "N."

B: *Pores:* are they open or tight?

If open, you have oily skin. Are they tight? You have normal skin.

Invisible? Dry skin.

C: *Chin:* do you have pimples or whiteheads? (A pimple is a red bump filled with pus, usually with a white point. A whitehead is a white-colored blemish deep underneath the skin.) If yes, write "O." All clear, write "N."

D: *Hairline:* any pimples? If yes, oily skin. Any flaking? If yes, dry skin.

E: *Cheeks:* look for pimples, blackheads and wide-open pores—they all mean oily skin. If you have rough, red or flaky skin with no visible pores—your skin is dry.

If you found you have normal or dry skin, there is a way to tell whether your skin is dry or not. Check for flakiness and redness around the nose. If your skin is flaky, it's dry. If not, then it's normal.

Don't be surprised if you have a combination skin, which your drawing will clearly reveal. This is important to determine. You cannot judge your skin by one section.

Now take a Touch Test: Wash your hands and dry them well. Touch your forehead with your index finger. Is your finger now shiny? This means you have oily skin. The skin should feel soft. If it doesn't, this means you have dryness.

HOW TO CLEANSE YOUR FACE PROPERLY

Mother will inspect your fingernails, look behind your ears and ask if you've brushed your teeth, but she seldom teaches you how to clean your skin properly.

Knowing your skin type is essential to this process, and each requires its own cleansing routine:

For Dry Skin:

When you wake up in the morning use a light lotion without alcohol or a water-soluble cleansing cream. Clean in a circular motion—gently: don't rub or scrub—then rinse with cool water and pat dry. Apply moisturizer to cheeks and forehead.

Before bed at night use a light cleansing cream to soften and remove makeup, and follow the steps above.

For Oily Skin:

When you wake up in the morning use astringent to clean your face until the last cotton piece is completely clean. Don't miss your hairline. DO NOT USE RUBBING ALCOHOL as astringent, because it is far too strong for your skin. If your skin is very oily, choose a lotion with some alcohol content. This will reduce oils and fight bacteria. Use the best skin astringent you can afford—it doesn't have to be the most expensive one on the market, but it shouldn't be the cheapest either.

(Astringent is often called toner, cleansing lotion or tonic by various makers.)

Also use astringent on your chest, shoulders and back—treat them just as you do your face. If you can't reach your back, get some help. People with oily skin usually have blackheads on their backs, so keep those pores clean! If you do break out on your chest or back, clean with astringent twice a day, and once a week, soak in a tub, apply drying mask wherever blemishes plague you, then rinse it off in the shower. If you ever inadvertently open a blemish by scrubbing too hard, apply hydrogen peroxide to the blemish with cotton for two minutes.

Before bed at night use a light cleansing cream to remove your makeup; then use the astringent until the cotton comes clean. Clean cotton equals clean skin.

For Combination Skin:

When you wake up in the morning clean the oily parts of your skin with astringent as prescribed above. Then rinse your face with cool water. Moisturize by using a spatula to remove a small amount from the jar, place it in your palm and then apply with clean fingertips. (This keeps the product fresh.)

Before bed at night cleanse your skin with light cleansing cream, then apply astringent to oily areas only. If you have very dry skin in the dry areas, use only water-soluble cream. Apply drying preparation to any blemishes.

For All Skin Types:

Every morning use an eye cream. Apply with fingertip, dot gently, then pat off excess with tissue.

Cleansing products with granules in them should not be used every day. If you have oily skin and blackheads, you will need the abrasive action of the granules for deep cleaning once or twice a week, but too abrasive a cleanser can open up blemishes and cause infection or make your skin red and sore and spread infection. In choosing a cleanser with granules, pick a cream-based product, not just loose grains. This will be less abrasive to your skin. Use only on the offending areas. Also avoid abrasive cleaning pads; they scratch skin and break capillaries.

OTHER TREATMENTS

Moisturizing

A moisturizer is an emulsion that keeps moisture from seeping out of your skin by forming a barrier across it. Moisturizers soften your skin, alleviate dryness and tightness, and help it to retain water. They form a shield to help protect it. If your skin has a lot of natural oil, that oil will protect your skin. If you tend toward dry skin, you probably need help from a jar or tube. Always use a spatula to remove moisturizer from a jar to keep it free of contaminants; fingertips, even if just washed, usually have bacteria on them. Shift the moisturizer from spatula to palm, and using your fingertips, gently work it upward into the skin of your face and neck. You can refrigerate your moisturizer if you don't use much at a time, transferring it to a smaller jar for daily use or travel. This keeps creams fresher longer and avoids the risk of fast spoilage on the shelf. A moisturizer should have a shelf life of a year to a year and a half.

Steaming

For any skin other than sensitive skin, *steaming* is a very effective treatment to be practiced every week to ten days. The heat rising with the steam will open pores and soften the top layer of skin so you can clean out impurities and oils, and allow the pores to breathe a little fresh air. To make your own facial steam baths:

1. Boil water in a pot.
2. Put a heaping tablespoon of loose camomile tea leaves into the boiled water. Remove from heat.
3. Lean over the water and tent yourself in with a large bath towel. Steam should bathe your face.

BEFORE you begin your steaming, put a little cream on your face, except on your nose and chin. NEVER steam a dry face. When the vapor stops rising, your treatment is over.

After the steaming, you MUST use a mask to close up your pores or they will pick up dirt. There are various types available, depending on your skin type and needs.

Remove the mask with cotton and cold water. Pat your face dry.

Masks

Masks come in many formulas to do different jobs: stimulate circulation, soften skin, tighten skin, absorb oils and exfoliate dead cells from the skin's surface. No matter what type of skin you have, there is a right mask for you. Make sure you read the directions and follow them to the letter.

Choose your mask by your skin's needs. Dry skin will always need moisturizing masks; oily skin needs the drying aspects of clay. Combination skins will require the use of two *different* masks. Put a mask on clean skin (always after steaming), then sit back and relax for the five to twenty minutes it takes the particular product to do its work. Close your eyes, put your feet up and think beautiful thoughts. Then wash the mask off in cold water and pat your skin dry. Never put a mask over your eyelids—or too close to your eyes. And don't forget your neck if you have dry skin.

If you have *dry* skin, use a mask every seven to ten days. Choose a mask to MOISTURIZE.

If you have *oily* skin, use a mask once or twice a week—but no more. (Summer may call for the twice-a-week treatment.) Choose a mask that ABSORBS OIL.

If you have *combination* skin, buy TWO masks, one for each type of skin, and use them where needed. It takes a bit of patience, but you'll never forgive yourself if you don't do this right. Give yourself this double-whammy treatment every week or so. If your oily patches are extra bothersome, treat them every three or four days, alternating the double treatment with the oily treatment.

If you want to treat yourself like *royalty*, give your *hands* a moisturizing treatment after you've treated your face. All skin types will benefit, especially *dry* skin. After you apply hand cream, put your hands into cheap cotton gloves or pot-holder mitts (line each pot holder with a baggie to keep both hands and mitts clean) and relax for ten to twenty minutes. Rinse with warm water and apply light hand lotion. Your feet will enjoy the same treatment too!

YOU ARE WHAT YOU EAT

One of the basic facts of beauty is that the food you consume shows up in the condition of your hair, your nails and your skin. No skin cream, treatment or lotion can give your skin the good looks that reflect good health—and that comes from within.

You don't need to be a nutritionist to know what foods are good for your skin, nor do you have to have one of those mimeographed charts from your doctor to tell you which ones are enemies. There's no such thing as a "do's and don'ts" list, because when you eat a healthful, well-balanced diet, you can have a little of any type of food without causing damage to your skin.

Every meal should include one food from each of the four food groups.

Food Groups

Vegetable/Fruit	*Fiber*	*Dairy Products*	*Protein*
green leafy veggies	grain/cereal	milk/cheese	meat
root veggies	pasta		poultry
yellow veggies	rice		fish
citrus fruits	whole-grain breads		beans
soft fruits	(not refined		nuts
berries	white breads)		

The foods are classified according to the types of nutrients they contain, and you should eat amounts from each of the groups —without eating too much. While milk is a good protein source, it is also high in fat. A healthful combination of foods should always include plenty of fiber, and you should cut back on fats, oils, sugar and salt. Avoid excessive amounts of caffeine, alcohol and pickled and smoked foods. (These have all been linked to cancer.)

You should drink plenty of water, preferably bottled or purified, at meals and in between. (See page 37.)

Use common sense in choosing specialty foods—have wine, spicy foods, fried foods, candy, soft drinks and junk foods infrequently and in small amounts.

Eat real foods rather than artificial versions. If you insist on sugar, use the real thing (or honey) rather than a chemical substitute. But don't overdo.

If you're thirsty, avoid soft drinks (especially diet ones) and iced tea (iced tea in quantity will turn your teeth yellow), and drink bottled water or fruit juice mixed with club soda.

Prolonged fasting without a doctor's supervision is not safe. When you fast, the lack of nutrients can cause your skin to dry out or break out. Remember, if you are watching your weight, the idea is to cut down—not cut out.

If you are not eliminating regularly because of constipation, it will affect your skin. Roughage is a good solution to this problem. Try a breakfast of ¼ to ½ cup bran (the health-food-store kind, not the commercial mixed variety) with skim milk, and drink a lot of water.

Bumps on your face, especially around the mouth, without heads (like a rash) can be caused by stomach problems, nerves or something internal. (See page 58.) The best way to cure this type of skin reaction is to get to the root of the emotional problem and to cope with whatever is causing the anxiety. More exercise often helps to diffuse stress and clear the skin as well.

You may find yourself in a situation where it's difficult to eat a balanced meal. You may be forced to grab whatever food you can or rely on fast foods and junk foods to get you through the day. Invariably this haphazard kind of diet leads to skin trouble. If you're at camp, away at college, in the armed forces or at the mercy of institutional cooking, try some of these tips:

■ Eat whatever foods in the cafeteria line are the freshest. Make a meal out of the salad if need be. Avoid canned and pre-fab foods.

■ Don't try to hide the taste of the food with gravy, ketchup or sauces. They're fattening and they may cause a skin breakout.

■ Stay away from candy machines and vendors who sell potato chips, corn chips, popcorn and the like. If you must have popcorn, make your own in a hot-air popcorn machine and skip the salt and butter.

■ If you have oily skin, avoid animal fats. Butter, milk, yogurt, ice cream and especially cheese are harder to digest and may cause oily skin to break out. And simply cutting back on animal fats may clear up your skin dramatically. This is not a universal remedy, and it will take six to eleven weeks before you see results, but it is well worth the try.

■ Too many vitamin pills (especially A, E and B) may cause skin to break out. A daily multi-vitamin tablet should be all the supplement you need. Remember, vitamins are not a panacea, nor a substitute for a healthy diet. Too much of a good thing can indeed be bad news.

■ Spicy foods and shellfish often cause people to break out, as do acids like those in tomatoes or citrus fruits, even in coffee or wine. Try eliminating them from your diet for six to eleven weeks.

■ Drink lots of bottled water.

THE FOOD TEST: To see if your skin is reacting to something you've eaten, drop a suspect item from your diet without changing anything else. Wait and see what happens. Allow at least two weeks. Don't change everything at once, because then you won't know which item caused the breakout.

WATER, WATER EVERYWHERE

Water is the most essential nutrient your body can get. You can go without food, but you *cannot* do without water. Unfortunately, most people think of it only as a means to wash down a vitamin pill. Even if they are thirsty, they'll drink a liquid other than water. That old textbook rule about eight glasses a day does not mean six glasses of cola and an iced tea or two; pure, clean water is imperative for a healthy body and glowing skin.

■ Thirst is not a good indication of water needs. Drink six to eight glasses a day, whether you are thirsty or not.

■ Avoid ice water or extremely cold water.

■ Drink tap water only if you know the water in your area to be safe. When traveling (even within the United States), drink bottled water. Remember, ice cubes are made from tap water, so it's best to avoid them unless you make your own with bottled water.

■ Do not worry about "water weight"—you will lose it naturally. DO NOT rely on diuretics—this is very dangerous. Reducing your consumption of salt and sugar and refined flours will help combat water weight.

■ Space out your water drinking through the day—don't go for broke in one or two sittings. If you drink an eight-ounce glass before each meal, you will eat less.

■ Drink your last glass of water one hour

before bedtime; otherwise you may be rudely awakened.

■ Tempted to snack? Have a glass of water instead.

■ If you are training for an athletic event or involved in a lot of sports activity, drink water forty-five minutes before and after your workout (drinking right before exercise can cause stomach cramps). You should replace the water you sweat off and still have eight glasses more.

CLIMATE COUNTS

Climate plays a big role in skin condition—especially for people who live in regions with sharply defined seasons. Even people in temperate zones have to watch for weather swings, but the more extreme the changes, the greater the strain on your skin.

Pamela was a Southern beauty who rarely had a skin problem throughout high school and college. Her skin was on the dry side, which helped keep it from breaking out, but this never posed a serious problem. Then she moved to New York for her first big modeling job. Before Christmas she was miserable. Her skin was flaky, her nose was red, her lips were always cracked and brittle and she was developing pimples around her hairline. When I first looked at her skin, it was hard to figure out why she had the signs of wind and weather damage while simultaneously suffering from pimples and whiteheads. Then she told me that to combat the dry skin, she was using a heavy French cream under her makeup. This greasy cream was causing the whiteheads around the hairline but was still not saving her skin from the ravages of winter winds.

If your skin is dry, in the winter you should take especially good care of it *without* moisturizing so excessively you create a new problem. Wear protective clothing—keep your head covered and a scarf around your face and neck. Always wear lipstick or lip balm. Even in summer, dry skin should be moisturized—but that doesn't mean putting suntan or baby oil on it. Use a sunblock or a moisturizer, and avoid sunbathing, which could dry your skin even more. Sunbathing is always a no-no because it dries the surface of the skin and traps the oils underneath, so that you end up with aging dry skin on the top layer and eruptions underneath.

As a general rule (no matter what your skin type), use a *stronger* cleanser in summer, because oil glands are more active then, and a *lighter* moisturizer. In winter, reverse.

If you have oily skin, in winter you'll still need to protect it with a *light* moisturizer. Use it as sparingly as possible; then use a mineral-water spray from one of those plant-spritzer bottles, and blot. This way you won't give your oily skin too much extra oil. In summer, avoid suntan oils, and carry astringent (cleanser lotion) with you so you can mop up every few hours or as your skin needs it. Buy the smallest-size plastic bottle available at the drug or dime store and put cleanser in it. Carry it with you, with some clean cotton balls in a baggie. Or pre-dip them and place in baggie. Then it will always be convenient to wipe away excess oils. Don't overdry the top layer of your skin with chemical treatments, as this will trap oil beneath it and cause clogged pores or bumpy skin.

For combination skin you must be careful in all seasons, because you'll always be *combining* several care techniques on different parts of your face.

If a skin problem persists for four to six weeks, get professional help. Don't wait for the seasons to change. Find out what's going wrong, why and what to do about it now.

Winter is the cruelest season, when it comes to your skin. You go in and out of doors, alternating between cold air and indoor heating. Indoor heating means you're locked in with little humidity and much dry heat, which will cause surface dryness even to oily skins. Freezing temperatures contract the blood vessels on the skin surface so that whatever oil your glands normally secrete is slowed down to a crawl. Even oily skin suffers. All skins need to change their winter cleansing and moisturizing routines. (See page 34.) Dry, flaky patches can make their way to your face—and other parts of your body as well—even if you have oily skin and even if that part of the body (elbows, legs, hands) is not exposed to raw cold air. Dry skin gets drier than ever as the moisture content of the air drops.

Summer may be easier on your body than winter, but too much sun can be more damaging to your skin than too much cold. (Unless you live in Siberia.) Nothing makes the skin age faster than sun wear. Though oily skin ages less quickly than dry skin, any skin type will suffer from too much sun, and fair skin can tolerate less abuse than olive. Tanning, be it outside by the pool or in one of those tanning parlors or booths, is extremely dangerous to the future health of your skin. Remember, there is no such thing as a healthy tan. You *can* get a little color without getting bronze.

Damage from sunning will not show up immediately, but once it has occurred, it is irreversible. Sun damage causes premature aging, and sun worshipers end up looking ten to fifteen years older than their true age. Sun damage can also cause white or brown spots, changes in pigmentation, skin cancer and so on. While the skin cancers can usually be removed, this is not something to take lightly!

Use a sunscreen or sunblock on all parts of your body that are uncovered, reapplying it every two hours and always after swimming. The fact that you are wearing a block does not mean your skin won't feel hot. If this sensation is bothersome, go indoors immediately, and apply a moisturizer. Wear sunglasses while outside, or goggles, and a sweatband. A hat or bandana offers sun protection for your hair; sun visors give eyes and face extra protection, especially those with a wide brim.

SCREEN THOSE RAYS

While moisturizers and makeup bases now come with sunscreens added, I recommend a full-strength sunscreen. Choose a gel or oil-free one if you have oily skin; a cream if you're dry. Then apply your base.

Before choosing a sunscreen, learn to read

two important letter codes: PABA and SPF.

PABA stands for para-aminobenzoic acid and is the most helpful of the sunscreens because it absorbs ultraviolet light B, the rays that burn your skin. Some sunscreens combine PABA and another chemical called benzophenone to cover a wider spectrum of light, offering even better protection. (Alone, benzophenones wash or sweat off easily and don't offer the same protection as PABA.)

While PABA is a chemical, SPF measures the amount of protection in a sunscreen or block. It stands for Sun Protection Factor and is based on how long the product will protect you from turning red. It's usually measured numerically, between 2 and 22; the higher the number, the more protection it offers. Fifteen is considered high, but you may find ratings up to 20. SPF of 8 or less is a sunscreen (you'll get more color); 9 or more is a block. Different skin types need different types of sunblock, but here's a general idea of how SPF can help you pick a product that will protect you from burning, while allowing a little healthy color to come through.

Skin Type	SPF
very fair never tans burns easily	15 or more
tans a little	15–8, gradually moving lower over the summer
rarely burns tans	8–6
rarely burns tans splendidly	6–4
never burns dark or olive	4

SUN ANNOUNCEMENT

Certain drugs can cause your skin to become more sensitive to the sun—to develop a photosensitivity. If you are taking a medication, ask your doctor. Birth-control pills, sulfa drugs, tetracycline and tranquilizers may make your skin more sensitive to sun.

For maximum protection use sunblock when walking or driving. It is possible to get a burn through glass, so protect while in the car.

BATHS, SHOWERS, BIDETS

I can think of few things more relaxing than a hot bath—or worse for your skin. Give yourself a hot bath only as a treat. Limit yourself to one or two a week. Other bath tips:

- Aim for warm rather than hot water, especially if you have dry skin;
- DO NOT add fragrance or oils, as they can irritate sensitive tissues and cause gynecological infections. Use such products *after* you emerge;
- If you shave your legs in the tub, wait until you have soaked for a few minutes so skin is softer and pores are open;
- Blot off water when you get out of the tub—don't rub-a-dub-dub. Moisturize with a body cream before you dry off completely.

Brief showers are better for your skin.

- Keep water cool or warm rather than *hot*;
- DO NOT shower several times a day if you can help it.

Remember the bidet! Most American homes do not have bidets, but the underlying principle still applies—you don't have to soak in order to clean up. Wash your private parts daily with a mild, unscented soap. Underarms and feet need daily washing too.

HEALTHY BODY SKIN

While few women like a nose that glows like Rudolph's, your body skin should have a slightly shiny look. Not greasy, but glowy. Wrinkles, defects and stretch marks will not show as readily when light reflects off this shimmer.

No matter what type of facial skin you have, your body skin can be a totally different type. Ashley has combination skin on her face, oily chest and shoulders and dry elbows, arms, thighs and buttocks! (She treats her two body skin types differently and is careful the body cream she uses on her thighs and buttocks never meets her shoulders and mid-back area.)

To get the body glow you want:

- Eat well; exercise daily;
- Use a gentle body brush (but not the rough rubber kind) rather than a loofah to exfoliate and aid circulation without pulling out hairs or damaging moles. (My friend Wayne makes his own out of tulle.) Skin should feel invigorated, not sore (This also improves circulation, which will help you shine prettily.);

■ If you have dry body skin, use body cream after bathing, while your skin is still moist; body cream is less expensive than products meant for the face, and usually comes in appropriately large containers.

■ Even if you have very dry skin, don't *smother* it with creams. Skin needs to breathe and perspire.

SKIN CHANGES IN PREGNANCY

Pregnancy causes many changes in the body, changes that can differ dramatically from person to person. Some women claim they glow when they are pregnant; others get their very first blemishes and eruptions. Some experience a darkening of the skin known as the "mask of pregnancy." They have no warning of this condition; suddenly they develop brown spots, or a stripe across the tummy or even a new skin tone. Sometimes you can prevent the change from occurring by using a sunblock when you are outdoors and by giving up sunbathing completely.

Blemishes during pregnancy are due to the hormones running around your constantly changing body. Because the skin is far more vulnerable to scarring while you are pregnant, it's important that you allow blemishes to heal naturally—so remember: hands off. Try changing your cleansing routine to one for oily skin and purchase a drying agent.

Many of the changes—including the darkening—are temporary, and your skin and body will return to normal after the baby is born. If you are breast-feeding, allow a little bit longer for your skin to return to normal; I've seen many women who have skin problems or sensitivities while they are nursing. Don't panic—enjoy your new baby, and you'll manage to cope with whatever changes come your way.

SKIN CARE FOR MEN

Men have the exact same skin types as women, so there is no reason a man shouldn't take care of his skin in the same way. Some men think it's macho not to do anything to enhance their looks. Many more are beginning to realize the health benefits of taking care of themselves. If you want to help the man in your life—be it a father, brother, boyfriend or husband—don't make an issue of skin care; just see if you can get him to try out a new routine and see how it works.

■ Suggest that he use your products—if you have the same skin type. (You can say something casual: "I just got this fabulous new cleanser I think you'll like.")

■ Buy him a gift.

■ Get him a gift certificate to a salon that treats men. Whatever you do, never embarrass him. Men are afraid you'll think they are sissies if they pay attention to their skin. But the intelligent man is doing the same thing an intelligent woman is doing—taking care of a good thing. Men should:

1. Use cleansing lotion according to skin type and avoid soap on the face.
2. Use a light moisturizer, unless they have acne. It should not be greasy or discernible to touch or sight.
3. Use a light under-eye cream during the day. (Yes, even men!)
4. Use cleansing lotion again at night.

If a man has a breakout, he should treat it with a drying preparation. Use a mask for blackheads. If he wears a beard, it can be made softer with the right shampoo and conditioner. (Many women get rashes and burns from their boyfriend or husband's beard. If you hurt—say something! I have even treated a woman with painful sores on her chin caused by beard burn.)

David suffered from a new outbreak of pimples almost every day. He thought he had incurable acne and learned to tolerate the condition, even though he was thirty-five and had had the problem since his teens. When Natalie fell in love with him, she was determined to do something about his badly troubled skin. She guessed correctly that Dave did not have acne, just a bad case of oily skin that he was ignoring. It took her almost a year to persuade him to come to my salon so I could look at his skin. Yet within six weeks after my seeing him, his complexion was almost clear—thanks mainly to an effective cleansing program. All those needless years of embarrassment and pain . . .

PREVENT PREMATURE AGING

How you age is partially a genetic matter. But there are several Get Smart techniques that will help you look better longer:

- Avoid sunbathing;
- Always use a sunscreen or sunblock when outdoors—even on cloudy days;
- Don't smoke—it's bad for your insides and it ages your face and skin;
- Keep alcohol intake at a minimum;
- Keep your weight within three to five pounds of its ideal level throughout your lifetime;
- Get adequate rest, relaxation and sleep;
- Avoid harsh cleansers;
- Use proper moisturizing techniques for your skin type;
- Moisturize your neck daily;
- Eat well-balanced meals;
- Establish correct posture;
- Stay away from medication and drugs as much as possible;
- Use a humidifier in winter;
- Avoid saunas.

UNHOLY SMOKE

Smoking creates squint lines around the eyes from the smoke drift. The pursed lips used to hold the cigarette and puff create tiny lines around the mouth. And the smoke affects skin color. NO SMOKING!

SKIN CARE AND SPORTS

More and more people understand the importance of exercise and sports to good health, and as a result, more people include a daily workout in their lifestyle. The only problem with exercise (besides the occasional charley horse) is that it causes you to perspire. Perspiration is vital, because it releases waste from within. It is a cleansing process for both the body and the skin. However, allowed to sit on your skin for hours, perspiration may clog your pores and cause its own skin problems. It is possible to be allergic to your own perspiration and actually develop redness or a rash from it.

If you go to exercise class, go with clean skin and no makeup base. *Do* apply lots of eye cream. Keep your hair pulled off your face in a ponytail, or with combs, a sweatband or scarf. (If you use a sweatband, be sure to wash it every day.) Immediately after class, clean your skin before you leave the gym. If you have dry skin, apply a light moisturizer.

If you swim, remember that your whole body gets dry, so use a rich cream all over at night. Your skin will get old and rough fast if you are not careful. Before swimming, use a lubricant on your face. If you have dry skin, it will be protected. If your skin is oily, use a light moisturizer rather than a thick cream. However, if you have acne, don't use a moisturizer at all. If you are swimming outdoors, use a sunblock or a sunscreen instead of moisturizer. Also be sure to care for your hair properly, because the water and chlorine will dry and damage it. Wear a swim cap, or pin your hair up and don't get it wet! Use extra hair conditioner afterward.

If you jog, before you set one foot on the ground, make sure your skin is clean and you have dabbed eye cream around your baby-blues (or baby-browns). If you're jogging in the sunshine, make sure you wear a sunblock or sunscreen, and use a visor to protect the delicate skin around your eyes. In your pocket—or in a money belt, if your jogging suit has no pockets—carry some cotton soaked in astringent in a Baggie. If you start to sweat, or jog along a roadway, dab away the dirt immediately. If your skin is very dry, jog with a light moisturizer on your face and neck. When you get home, cleanse your skin and apply a nourishing cream, massaging it upwards with your fingertips; then apply warm cotton compresses to ensure that it penetrates. Make certain you wash out your sweatband after each use.

If you play tennis, use a visor, which is better than a hat because it can be pulled farther down on your face to give you more protection from the sun. Use a sunscreen or sunblock on all parts of your body that are exposed; wear sunglasses and a clean sweatband. Sun-sport enthusiasts are often candidates for skin cancer, so make sure your skin is well protected. Keep your hair off your face (you'll see better, too).

If you ski, realize that you are setting yourself up for many types of skin abuse—from sun, glare and wind—so heavy protection is needed. For water skiing, use a moisturizer with a sunscreen in it and an eye cream. For snow skiing, beat dry skin with a heavier moisturizer and a milder cleanser. If you warm up after skiing with a hot bath, be sure to moisturize your whole body afterward. Take mini-containers of sunscreen and lip balm with you on the slopes. Place them in the zippered pockets of your ski attire; reapply on the lift.

For all outdoor sports, apply moisturizer to your skin first, wait five minutes, then apply sunblock or sunscreen. Moisturizer with a sunscreen already in it is not sufficient. Also use an eye cream, protect your lips with a cream or gloss, and wear sunglasses or goggles. When you come in, clean your skin thoroughly and use a nourishing treatment.

Don't forget that neck and hands need protection indoors and out.

SKIN CARE AND TRAVEL

Before leaving on a trip, always think of where you are going and how the climate there could affect your skin. If you go, for example, from a town in the midwest with relatively clear air to New York or Boston, be prepared with a stronger cleanser.

Air travel, and the lack of moisture in the cabin, is very drying to the skin, hands and eyes, and it is best to travel with skin free of makeup, and especially eye makeup if possible. This cuts down chances of arriving with sore, red and tired eyes.

It's a good idea to disappear into the ladies' room during the flight to clean your skin (bring a Baggie with pre-moistened cotton balls), then apply a mask if the flight is long enough. Rinse off and apply moisturizer.

Always travel wearing a generous amount of eye cream. I like to carry hand cream along and apply during the flight. I have never understood why the airlines persist in passing out boiling hot towels (drying) soaked in alcohol-perfume (drying) when the passengers are already suffering from lack of moisture.

Lastly, if you work on a plane, be sure to buy a heavier moisturizer just for your working hours—it will help.

RULES OF THE SKIN GAME

Here are some of the skin commandments my mother passed on to me.

Do's:

1. Do understand that your skin-care program will be successful only if you follow it with religious commitment.
2. Do cleanse your face as often as possible, with the cleanser recommended for your skin type.
3. Do protect your skin during the day with the proper moisturizer. (Unless you have acne.)
4. Do apply drying preparations when necessary.
5. Do keep your hair away from your face, especially at night.
6. Do keep your scalp in good condition. Flakiness or excessive oil can irritate your skin, especially at the hairline.
7. Do protect your skin from sun- and windburn.
8. Do avoid foods that you find irritate your skin.
9. Do drink lots of water. (Preferably bottled—these days tap water isn't always healthful.)
10. Do pay attention to good nutrition.
11. Do get as much rest as possible.
12. Do have your skin re-evaluated periodically as its needs change throughout the year.
13. Do spend as much time cleaning your skin as you do applying makeup.

Don'ts:

1. Don't squeeze your blemishes.
2. Don't scrub your skin: that's irritating. Especially avoid any scabbed areas. Scabs must be allowed to fall off naturally. If they are removed prematurely a scar can occur.
3. Don't use perfumed skin-care preparations.
4. Don't try to hide blemishes or problem areas under makeup.
5. Don't use hair spray.
6. Don't experiment with your friends' makeup.
7. Don't apply foundation with your fingertips; use clean sponges.
8. Don't dry out the top part of your skin without treating what's underneath.
9. Don't use washcloths or towels on your face; they're abrasive. Also, laundry detergents or bleaches can be in the fabric and may irritate your skin.
10. Don't put moisturizer on blemished areas.

Three

Problem Skin

Depending on age, heredity, climate, health care and the kind of makeup you use, your skin will continue to change throughout your life. It takes work to make that change for the better—first to clear up problem skin; then to protect it from damage, and to lessen the effects of age and stress.

You should know your skin's worst enemies:

- The magnifying mirror
- Your hands

You needed your magnifying mirror just once in your life: it helped you in the previous chapter in your overall assessment of your skin type. Now take that mirror and place it directly in the garbage can. If you don't get rid of it, you will spend all your spare time scrutinizing your skin and picking on pores that are better left alone. No one else sees you through a magnifying glass, so don't create trouble.

Likewise, your hands may be very becoming to the rest of your body, but they can do serious damage when they start to wander around your face, squeezing and pressing at whatever imperfection they encounter. Even unconsciously allowing your fingers to meander over your face can deposit infection-causing bacteria.

Over 99 percent of the people I have worked with or interviewed admit to picking at their skin at one time or another. Even those who know they shouldn't still do. Remember: a pimple will heal by itself without a scar; but if you squeeze, the pimple will not disappear as quickly and may well leave a trace. Maybe your skin won't scar the first two or three times, but believe me, sooner or later that poor little pore won't be able to take the abuse anymore. It may bounce back into shape with a lot of elasticity when you are young, but repeated irritations will cause permanent damage.

If you have a pimple that needs opening—don't touch it! Do yourself—and your complexion—a favor and see a professional cosmetician and let him or her do the deed. Keep the area clean, but don't dig at it. Don't use hot compresses, either. Many people wrongly assume they can release the pus behind a pimple with a steaming compress. I had an actress client who thought she could dissipate a blemish with a compress and ended up with a burn that was far worse than the original pimple! Get professional help and keep your hands to yourself!

A BLEMISH IS BORN

I had a client who had truly terrible skin. She freely admitted that she was guilty of skin abuse. What I didn't find out until years later, however, was that she picked her skin because she was so unhappy at home. Every night she would fight with her parents and then go into the bathroom and take out her frustrations on her face. As soon as she moved into her own apartment, her skin "miraculously" cleared up. It turned out she was happier away from her parents, and she stopped attacking her skin. This is a case where someone with oily skin created an "acne" skin by squeezing and infecting her pores.

If you have pimples that need to be opened, go to a good, licensed cosmetician who knows how to do it. Among the best-trained are those who have studied in the Eastern Bloc countries, Holland or Israel. They have devoted years to the study of skin problems. They often work with a doctor, performing deep cleaning and removing blackheads, whiteheads and pimples. French- or English-trained cosmeticians won't know how to do the kind of deep cleaning that's needed in pimple draining unless they have studied elsewhere. (In France or England, most facials consist of a mask and a massage without deep-pore cleansing.)

If you cannot find a qualified cosmetician in your city, let the blemish alone. It *will* heal naturally. Instead, do what you can at home. (See page 55 and *ignore* the pimple.) While your skin will slowly replace itself over a period of years, you have to live with your face every day. Don't jeopardize it with overanxious hands and a magnifying mirror insatiable in its demands for microscopic purity. Remember, a scar is damaged tissue, and though it may fade with time, it will never completely disappear.

RECOGNIZING AND LABELING PROBLEM AREAS

Once you've taken my Telltale Nose Test (see page 25), you'll be attuned to your skin's first trouble signals. Usually, the area around the nose and the top of the cheeks is the first to develop blackheads or oily patches. Then, in no particular order, standard problem areas usually include:

The chin (in particular, the cleft area of the chin);

The hairline (from ear to ear, anyplace—everyplace);

Forehead (dead center, of course, where everyone is looking);

Cheeks (usually right under the cheekbones where the skin is a little softer).

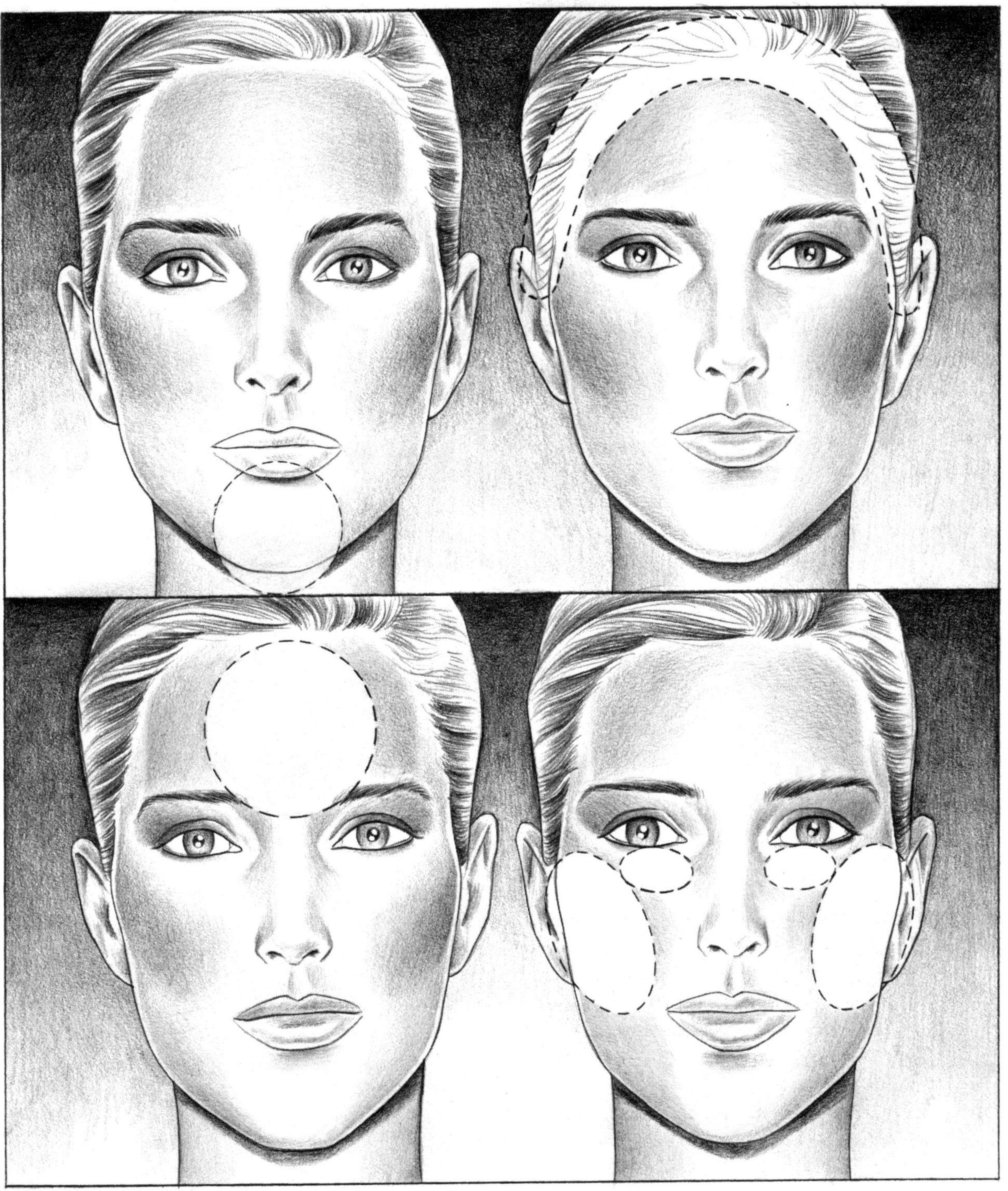

You can tell a specific area is a problem when you get two pimples there within a two-week period. Lightning rarely strikes twice in the same place; ditto pimples.

If you get a second blemish in the same area, then you have a problem that needs attention.

If you decide not to get help right away, watch the "problem area" for a couple of months (two, no more than three). You may want to treat yourself to some topical drying treatments, but beware of overdrying your skin. If you continue to have blemishes in the same region, you need professional help. Time will not cure your condition.

Of course, if your problem area develops during a pregnancy or is active only when you have (or are expecting) your period—disregard the foregoing advice. There's not much you can do about these breakouts because they are caused by changing hormones.

If you can't get to a skin expert, don't panic. Instead:

- Use a stronger cleansing lotion;
- Watch your diet carefully;
- Use a good topical drying agent;
- Don't put moisturizer on the skin in the war zone;
- Keep your hands *away* from your face!

When you do have recurring problems, do yourself the favor of getting help. Parents often tell you that irritations and breakouts are something you will outgrow, but I must disagree. If you are embarrassed or suffering socially because you have problem skin, you will also suffer emotionally. And this will affect your entire outlook on life and the way your personality develops in the upcoming crucial years.

DO I NEED HELP?

To help you decide if you need to see a professional, circle Yes or No after these statements:

1.	My skin is always broken out in one place or another.	*Yes No*
2.	My skin always breaks out in the same place.	*Yes No*
3.	My skin breaks out only before my period.	*Yes No*
4.	If I pick my skin, it gets better immediately.	*Yes No*
5.	Before a big date, my skin always breaks out.	*Yes No*
6.	When I'm nervous or tense, my skin breaks out.	*Yes No*
7.	My skin reacts to certain foods.	*Yes No*
8.	Other members of my family have had acne.	*Yes No*
9.	I perspire a lot during sports or exercise.	*Yes No*
10.	I wear a lot of makeup all the time.	*Yes No*

Now let's go through these responses together and see if you are a candidate for the experts.

1. If your skin is always broken out, you definitely need help.

2. If your skin breaks out in the same place and this breakout is not connected to menstruation or pregnancy, you need professional help.

3. If your skin breaks out only before your period, and clears up afterward, you do not need help. Try a stronger cleanser two weeks *before* your period. If you use a drying agent, follow the directions, because there are two different kinds—those applied directly to a blemish and those for blemish-prone areas.

4. If you pick your skin only once (a mistake) and it clears up without infection or another blemish forming, you still haven't done the right thing. You may be lucky at first, but before you ruin your skin you could benefit from professional advice.

5. Nerves may be making those blemishes appear, so professional help cannot prevent the breakout. But seek expert help for an analysis. Routine cleansing of pores is good and advisable because it cleans out small impurities before they enlarge.

6. Nerves and hormones both affect your skin, but a skin-care expert can help you. Have your gynecologist check your hormone levels; perhaps exercise or a fast-paced sport will help your nerves. Or you just might need a series of chats with a psychologist or psychiatrist.

7. If your skin reacts to certain foods, you don't need a cosmetician to tell you to have the good sense to lay off.

8. Skin type is hereditary, so if acne or problem skin runs in your family, a cosmetician can help you control your skin type before a problem makes you truly miserable.

9. If you perspire a lot during sports, your skin may need special care. Indeed, do consult a cosmetician.

10. If you wear a lot of makeup, you could be clogging your pores and not cleansing properly. A cosmetician will give you a cleansing routine that will be a lifetime system for keeping your skin in good shape. (Or see pages 33–34 for my basic routine.)

Let me tell you the story of Allison. She had been having trouble with her skin since puberty. She begged her mother to allow her to get professional help. First, her mother said she was too young. A year later, she agreed to let her try some drugstore remedies. Finally, for Allison's sixteenth birthday, her mother agreed to let her come see me at the salon. Not only had she had to endure the misery of pimples, but she was envious of her cousin who was the same age and seemed to have perfect skin. Allison explained to me that her cousin did nothing special to take care of her skin but rarely had a breakout, while she worked as hard as she could to prevent her pimples but just couldn't seem to beat them. This put me in an awkward position—because once Allison named her cousin, I realized that the girl suffered from skin problems just as bad as Allison's and had evidently been coming to the salon in secret for the past three years!

The moral of the story is to get help when you first need it. *There's no reason to be miserable.* In your teen years, your skin problems will not come and go in a matter of months. Because it takes years for your body to evolve from child to adult, your skin may have several turbulent years. Professional help from the beginning will make you happier—and prettier.

A few blemishes are no big deal to parents. But they can be to young women and men. If you have an unusual mole, or eczema, or warts, you should go to see a dermatologist. If your skin is breaking out, treat it with the same respect. The expert you should see is a cosmetologist.

Why not a dermatologist?

A dermatologist is used to seeing medical cases: burn victims, allergy sufferers, victims of serious diseases which manifest themselves through skin rashes or disfigurements. A doctor may not consider a few pimples or a shiny nose a serious problem and may not give you the attention and care you deserve. Most dermatologists see their patients for five to fifteen minutes. They don't have the time to open each clogged pore. Many give their teenage patients medication to solve their skin problems. The medical journals I have read offer inconclusive evidence that such medications (particularly antibiotics) actually work.

Very often, a licensed cosmetician—a specialist without an M.D.—can help basic troubled skin. To this kind of professional, blackheads are a problem and a challenge.

Cosmeticians:

- Do prepare the skin before removing "impurities";
- Do allot at least twenty minutes to this part of the treatment alone;
- Do consider your dry skin and blackheads to be problems;
- Do soften the top layer of skin;
- Do NOT let you leave with oozing skin;
- SHOULD NOT use instruments that break the skin.

Of course, there are many bad cosmeticians and many excellent doctors. How do you know which avenue to pursue?

FINDING A COSMETICIAN

All major cities have cosmeticians who can give you good advice and who are trained to help your skin. If you live in a smaller city or rural area, there may not be a cosmetician available. In that case, a dermatologist or general practitioner will be able to help you with serious skin problems. But the doctor may not know about the more delicate aspects of skin care.

When you begin your hunt for a cosmetician, make sure she (or he) is licensed by the state and that the license is hanging in plain view. Don't be embarrassed to ask to see it. *Never* go to a person who is not licensed! Then find out how long the cosmetician has been working (Practice makes perfect) and something about her (his) background—especially international training. Generally, if she has been trained only in the United States, she has only a hairdresser's license and has not learned as much about skin as she ought to know. She has no formal education in deep cleansing and extraction, so it would be unwise to let her do these procedures.

References from friends are helpful, especially if you live in a city where there are several well-known salons. You may also have to invest in personal experimentation. Salons offer a variety of philosophies; you'll have to find the one right for you. Often you are simply more comfortable at one salon or with one certain cosmetologist than another.

WARNING: if the cosmetician asks you what kind of skin you have, get up and out of the chair and leave at once. And never go back. A true expert will know your skin type just by looking, touching and asking one or two significant questions.

SALON TREATMENTS

If you have problem skin and can afford a salon facial, I recommend it. Sometimes you can buy a series of facials at a saving. Always ask for special prices or packages. It

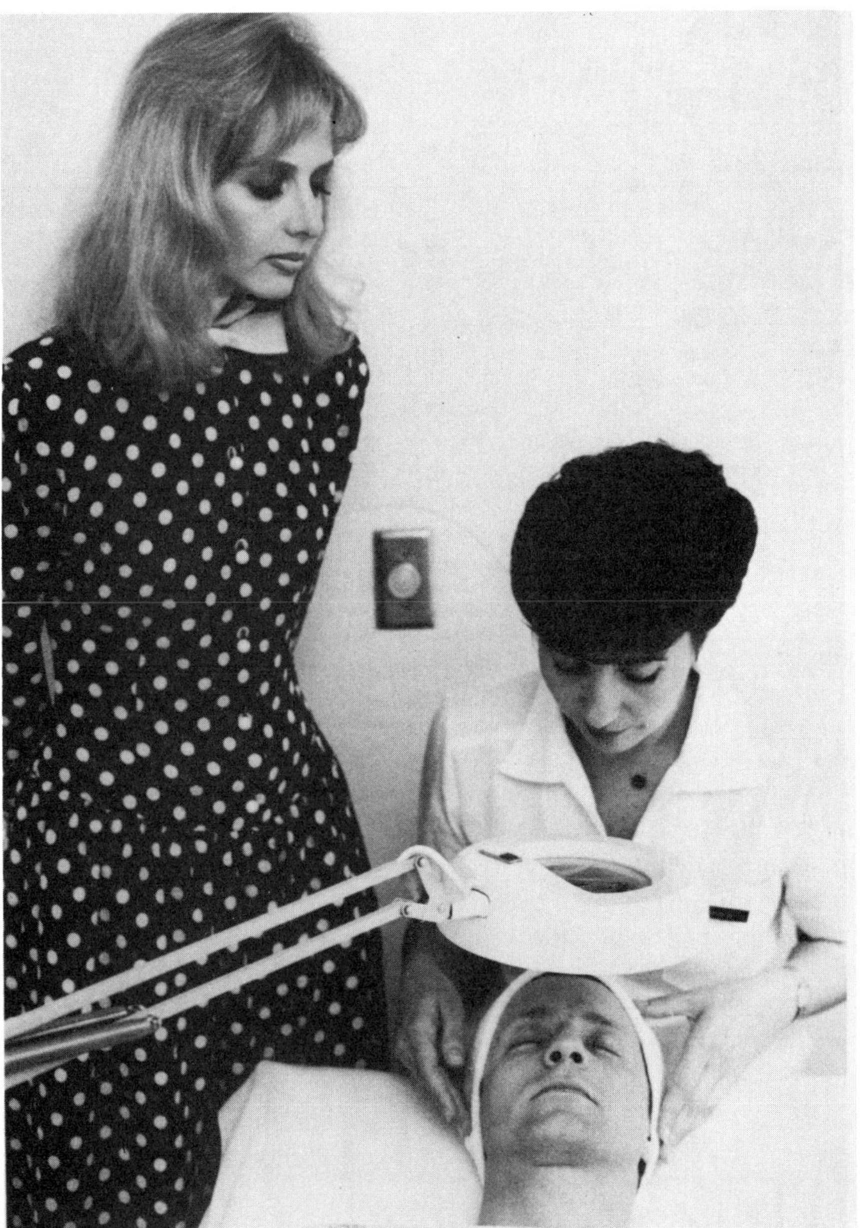

A salon facial starts with a skin analysis and a thorough deep cleaning.

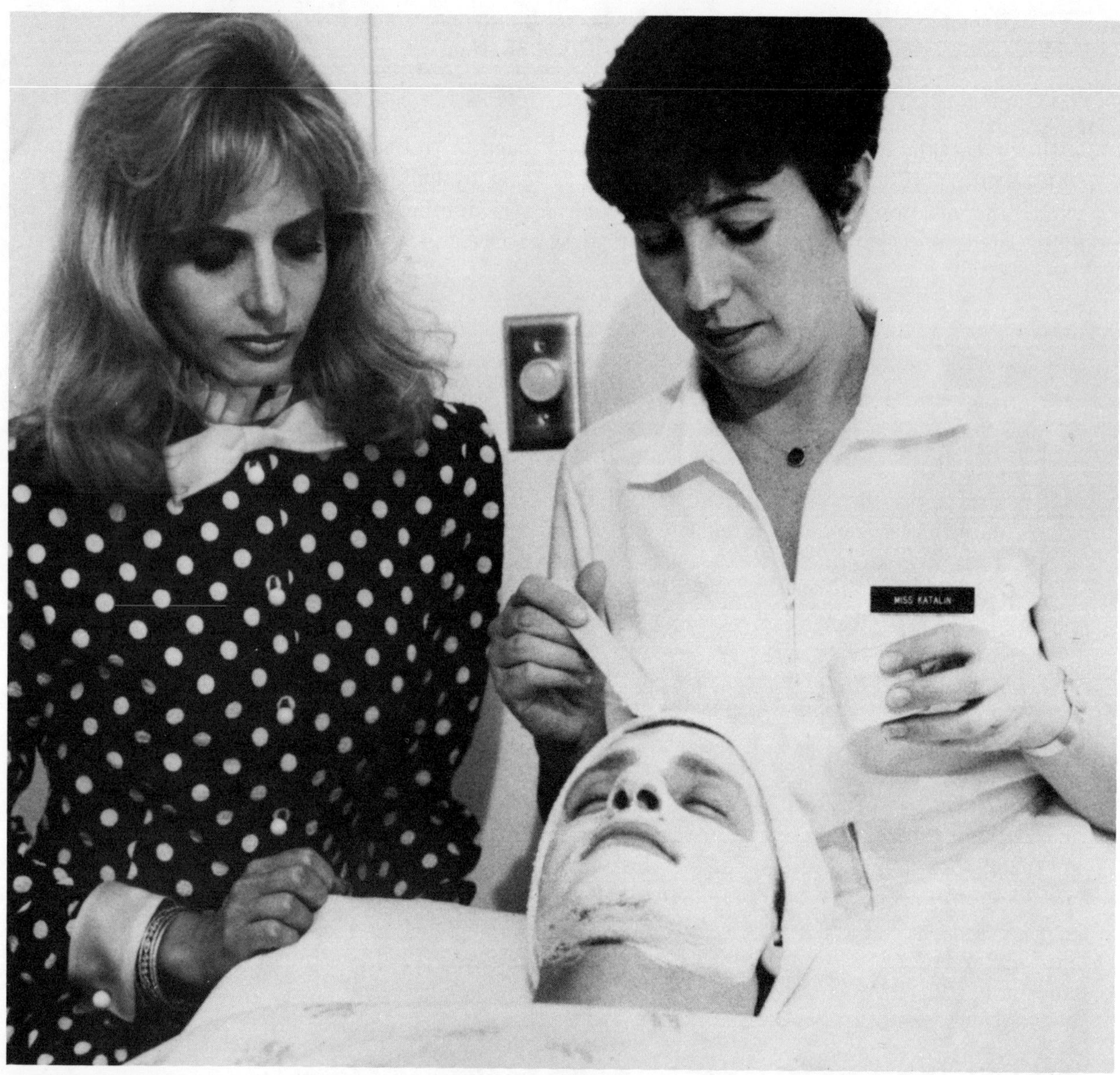

After the cleaning treatment a mask is applied to tighten pores and invigorate skin.

should take about six weekly facials to clear up a small problem, and then maybe one or two a month for maintenance. (If you have no problems, a facial every two to six months will ensure clean skin.) If you can have only two facials a year (Ask for gift certificates for your birthday and Christmas), go to a salon right before summer and again in the fall as the weather begins to change. Everyone should have a professional look at her skin once or twice a year.

Many salons sell their own cosmetics and skin treatments and will recommend that you buy them. You may even feel that the salon is being a bit pushy with its own products. If you liked the treatment and need help, start with the basics and build. Never run out and buy five new products *before* a facial—see what your needs are first. You can also schedule visits when your own inventory is depleted; that way you will get all the expert advice you need beforehand. Care products within a line are designed to work together, so generally, mixing and matching isn't the best idea. The cosmetician who works with you will know the line she works with and can best choose what she feels is most effective for your skin. If you trust her to do the delicate work of cleaning your face, you should trust her opinion on products and needs. But you should never feel pressured to buy. (If the sell is too strong and you don't know what to do, simply say, "I'd like to think about that. Thank you very much.")

Stay away from machine treatments—they damage skin.

Be prepared for a few days of healing after troubled skin has been cleaned.

BE YOUR OWN COSMETOLOGIST

If you do live in an area without a cosmetician or good skin-care salon, be your own skin-care counselor by following these steps:

- Keep your skin as clean as possible. That means cleansing three times a day, at least! Remember not to use soap and water. Soap will give your skin a tight feeling that can mislead you to think it's clean. Use a cleansing cream, then an astringent lotion. Then rinse with cool water. Do not leave the astringent on your skin! Keep astringent in a small plastic bottle, or pre-moisten cotton and place it in a Baggie, and take it to the office or school with you. Clean your skin often so that the oils don't sit on it and work their way into pimples.
- Remember, keep your hair off your face at night. Hair is a trap for smoke, pollution and bacteria which rub against the face while you are sleeping and cause blemishes and infections.
- And no matter what, never squeeze your skin!
- Don't try to cover a blemish by hiding it with foundation. This will only clog the pore and make matters worse. If you simply must wear foundation, use one that is oil-free.
- Don't wear moisturizer if you are broken out. Use only eye cream under your eyes.
- If you are tempted to play around with your skin, don't—apply a mask instead. You'll be doing your skin a favor and won't see the blemish you are dying to attack.
- If your work requires talking on the phone a lot, or you spend a lot of your after-school hours on the phone, clean the part of the receiver that touches your face and hair with rubbing alcohol daily to keep oils and bacteria from irritating your skin.
- Avoid homemade remedies you read about in magazines or see on television. Anything made in the kitchen should be eaten, not put on your skin. It's a waste of good food to grind up something from the refrigerator and place it on your face, and it does your skin absolutely no good, since the nutrients won't penetrate the skin.
- Don't touch your face often or sit in a position that has your hands supporting your face. This may be an unconscious habit you have to break. Let your neck hold your head up, not your hands. So many people tell me their hands never touch their face, and their cheek is resting on the palm of their hand even as we talk!

SKIN MEDICATIONS

When choosing a line of beauty treatments, you should have the opportunity to experiment in order to see what products work best on your type of skin. BUT: never use several lines of products at once, for two reasons: 1) You won't know which is the one that's working and which isn't doing anything, or is causing harm; and 2) You will dry out your skin with a chemical blitz and have side effects you'll have to deal with far longer than the life of the blemish.

Many times a good product is modestly packaged, but is just as effective. That's what counts. Don't be snowed by pretty packages or Big Sell ads in magazines. Ask your friends what works for them; experiment on your own.

"Over the counter" skin medications, those sold without a prescription, come in nice packages, make wonderful promises and are very attractive—especially to a person with a pimple. Buy them one at a time and use each product for three to six weeks to see if it helps. If you are not pleased with the result, toss the product out and start over. Most popular medications contain benzol peroxide, which works for some, but not all, people. Read the directions. Some say to apply them only to the blemish, others to blemish pore areas. The former claim to heal blemishes, the latter to control oiliness. Nothing should cause burning, peeling or flaking unless the instructions specifically say so. (If you have an allergic or bad reaction, write to the manufacturer and return the product.)

While there are burns and peels that are formulated to remove damaged skin so fresh cells can grow again, these products are not sold over the counter. Peeling is never desirable without a doctor's care. A medication may sting for a moment when it is applied, but if it continues to burn—discontinue use and call your doctor. Skin may turn red momentarily but should quickly return to normal.

ACNE VS. PROBLEM PIMPLES

Some people will have a more severe problem with their skin than an occasional breakout. These people usually suffer from acne. Unlike blemishes caused by hormones or diet or nerves, acne is a chronic condition that requires special treatment. You do not get it from eating chocolate or touching frogs. (It is hereditary, but you may develop it even if your parents did not suffer.) Although acne is more commonly found in teenagers, about 20 percent of its victims are over twenty-one. While acne cannot be prevented, it can be effectively treated by a professional skin-care expert. This is no time for you to practice medicine yourself or shy away from special attention. People who treat themselves and pick at their skin often end up with scars that last a lifetime. Remember, the pimples appear on the surface of your skin, but the causes lie beneath—the treatment has to be more than topical. Drying out your surface skin will not solve your problem. Acne is too serious a problem to conquer yourself, locked silently in your bathroom in front of the mirror.

MORE HOPE

Accutane is a new acne treatment—available in pills—that works on cystic acne. A doctor must prescribe the medication and will decide how many pills you take per day and how long. (Treatment ranges from a period of weeks to four months.) The pills are expensive and still experimental, but they have been approved by the FDA. Though the medication does have some side effects (dry eyes and skin, severely parched lips, joint pains), the treatment can be very effective for *severe* cystic acne. DO NOT take Accutane during pregnancy. DO NOT take while trying to become pregnant, or for at least three months before. Many years' experience with any new drug is required to ascertain all bad effects. Science will not have the total picture until enough users have been guinea pigs. However wonderful the results are, there may be dangerous side effects.

Birth-control pills do help some women in the control of hormonal acne and breakouts. However, the controversy over their relationship to cancer cannot be ignored. Get several opinions before you take these pills. If there is a history of cancer in your family, tell your doctor.

Collagen is a protein that is currently being added to skin-care and makeup products and is also used for reconstructive work on the face, whereby the collagen is injected to "fill in" wrinkles, slight deformities and even acne scars. The injections are done by either a qualified dermatologist (not all do them) or a plastic surgeon. Collagen injections are still very new and very expensive. The results may not last, and it's still too early to know if there are any adverse side effects. Products may contain either natural or synthetic collagen—the label will not tell you, but a good clue is the price—natural collagen will be much more expensive, and the product will require refrigeration. While there is some controversy over the effectiveness of collagen additives, the topical collagens do bind water, which helps to protect hair or skin.

ALLERGIES AND BODY CHANGES

Changes in your body can have a direct effect on your skin. Sometimes, such as before your period or when you are pregnant, you just have to grin and bear it. Other times, a breakout may be your body's way of telling you something is going wrong inside—either physically or psychologically. Allergies can cause many types of skin reactions and may take ages to isolate. Don't panic: you can do some of the sleuthing on your own; then you can see an allergist.

If you notice a sudden breakout, try to investigate its cause:

- Have you been eating three well-balanced meals a day or are you leaning toward junk food?
- Is your next period due soon?
- Are you under stress or tension?
- Have you been fasting?
- Have you used any new skin products lately?
- Have you been picking your skin?
- Are you taking any new medication?
- Do you take birth-control pills?
- Have you quit your exercise program?
- Do you snuggle with a furry pet?
- Are you getting the sleep you need?
- Are you drinking plenty of water?
- Have you had a fever?
- Does your winter coat have a fur collar?

Many things can cause a skin change. Take inventory; look for clues. If a body change is not causing your recent breakout, perhaps an external or topical problem is.

PSYCHOLOGICAL THRILLERS

We all know that the head and the heart are intimately connected, so while you may be eating right, getting plenty of sleep and exercise, and keeping your hands as far from your pimples as possible—you're still blemished! The doctor says there's nothing wrong with you; your mother says it's just hormones; your friends say you look "gross" and you just want to disappear.

Just as a person can think himself sick (as in psychosomatic illnesses), an emotional upset or psychological crisis can cause any number of health and skin problems. Take the case of Jill. Jill was deliriously happy to be marrying Kenneth—the man of her dreams. She had no questions, no qualms, and thought herself the calmest bride in the world. She had planned a simple family wedding so there was no big gala to worry about. Three days before the ceremony, Jill's normally good skin erupted in aggressive pimples. No matter what she tried, each day she noticed new eruptions. How could she look beautiful in her wedding picture, let alone on her wedding day?

Jill's face never did clear up before the wedding. Despite the simple nature of the ceremony, it was still an emotional experience, and Jill's nerves threw her regular body chemistry completely out of whack. Three days afterward, Jill was fine again. She had her wedding pictures touched up and has lived happily ever after—with the added knowledge that emotional pressures do indeed affect the skin.

Four

Hair

CROWNING GLORY

Instant impressions. What do you see? Hair first, then skin. Glorious hair leads curious eyes toward glowing skin. Hair and skin work hand in hand, so tackle them separately but conquer them together to maximize your beauty potential.

Your hair can look disastrous:

- because the cut is all wrong for your face, figure or capabilities
- before your period
- because you aren't taking the necessary time with it
- from chemical (like chlorine) and sun damage
- because of medication you are taking (Even birth-control pills affect the hair.)
- as a result of a fad diet, poor nutrition or haphazard eating habits
- from overprocessing—too much color and too many perms
- because of emotional stress
- as a result of illness
- because scalp problems are creating dandruff or flaking

Hair, like skin, reflects the overall health of its owner. They also interact: your hairline or scalp condition can cause blemishes at the perimeter of your face; long hair can cause breakouts on the neck and chin.

Good hair is the perfect frame for a healthy complexion. You wouldn't buy a painting by one of the masters and put it in a dime-store Plexiglas frame, would you? Nor would you put a poster in a frame meant to hang in the Louvre. Hair and skin should complement each other, setting the tone for your overall look. Once you have them under control, the rest of your beauty regimen will fall naturally into place.

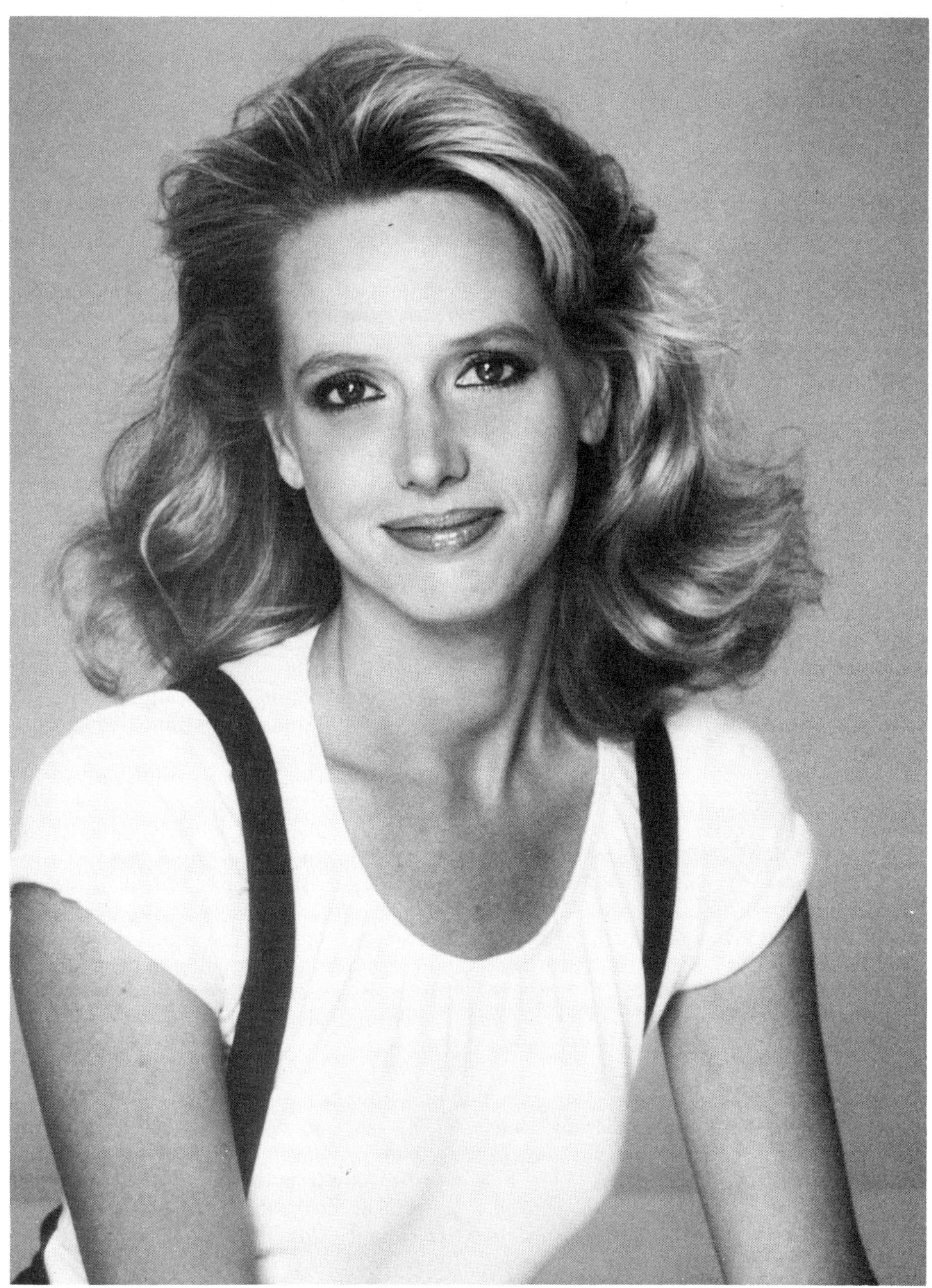

WASH AND DRY

You've been washing your hair since you were seven, but you are probably not washing it right. As a result, you may have split ends, chemical damage or flyaway hair that you blame on too much conditioner. Take some time out and start at the beginning. Proper shampooing is a learned art.

Remember:

1. Hair and scalp are related—you must wash both and treat them properly to have beautiful, healthy hair.

2. How often you wash your hair affects how often it *needs* to be washed. The more you wash—the more the oil glands in your scalp are stimulated—the dirtier your hair becomes. Europeans wash their hair twice a week, at most. Americans are so cleanliness-obsessed that many think it's imperative to wash their hair every day. That's just not so. Even if you believe in frequent washings, every other day is quite sufficient.

3. Don't use too much shampoo. It's expensive, it's a chemical and it will overclean —stripping too much oil from your hair. Dilute it with water. Shampoo is hard to get out of the hair and can settle on the scalp and cause "dandruff" or flakiness.

To shampoo:

1. Brush your hair first to eliminate tangles and snags.

2. Dilute the shampoo at a ratio of 1 teaspoon to ½ cup of water. If you have long heavy hair, a tablespoon of shampoo may be needed.

3. Thoroughly wet hair and scalp. The hair must be sopping wet for the shampoo to be effective. (Sudsing is no indication of a successful shampoo.) Never pour shampoo directly onto the scalp. If you have bangs that are more prone to oiliness than the rest of your hair, however, a direct dab of shampoo will help get them extra clean. Some rules do have exceptions!

4. Remember that the hair is not as dirty as the scalp, so manipulate your scalp with the fingertips of both hands. Work thoroughly, covering all parts of the hairline at the temples and nape of the neck, as well as the entire crown. Do not use fingernails or scratch at the scalp. It is not necessary to push your hair all around your head while shampooing; this will only cause nasty tangles. Just work on your scalp in a circular motion with the pads of your fingertips so that you can feel it moving. I never get tangles unless I'm at the hairdresser and the assistant doesn't wash my hair properly.

5. One sudsing is enough, even if you haven't shampooed in several days.

6. Rinse with warm (not too hot!) water, and lots of it. Rinse your scalp section by section to make sure you get all the shampoo out; then lift up your hair and get to rinsing the hair—all around your head. When you think your hair is clean, rinse thoroughly one more time.

7. After the warm rinse, use your conditioner. DO NOT apply conditioner to the scalp (This can cause flakiness or itching as well as oiliness). Conditioner goes on the ends of the hair. Apply from the ears down.

8. Now rinse with water that is gradually colder and colder until it's as cold as you can take it! This tightens the pores and gives the

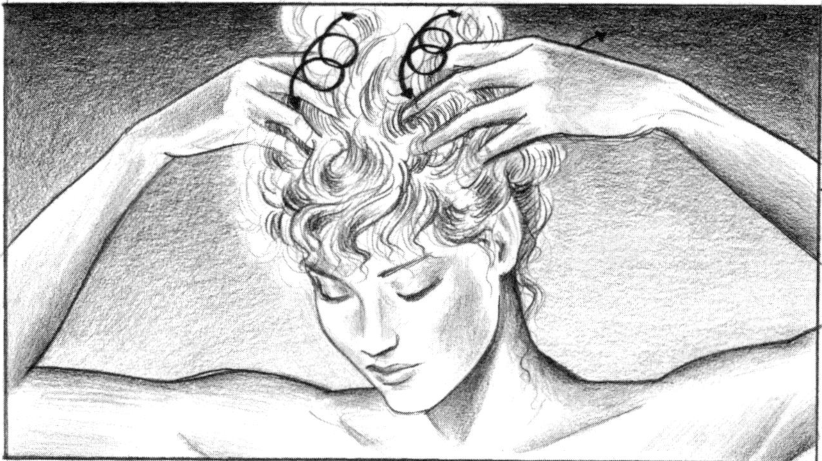

Gently use fingertips to work: crown,

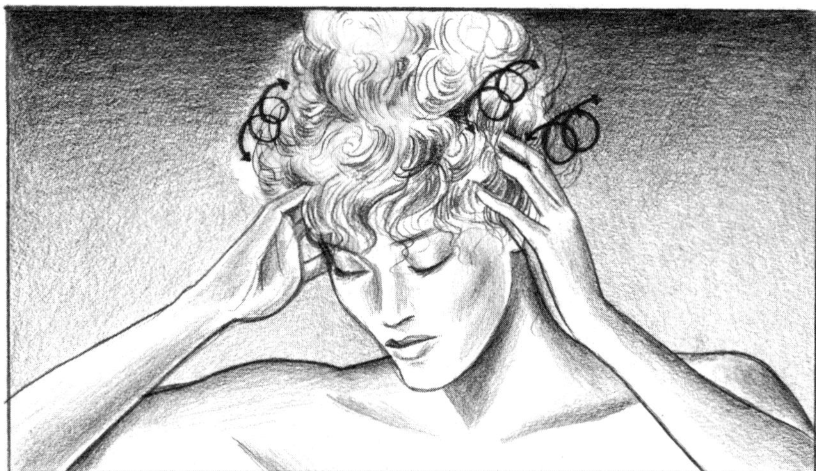

temples,

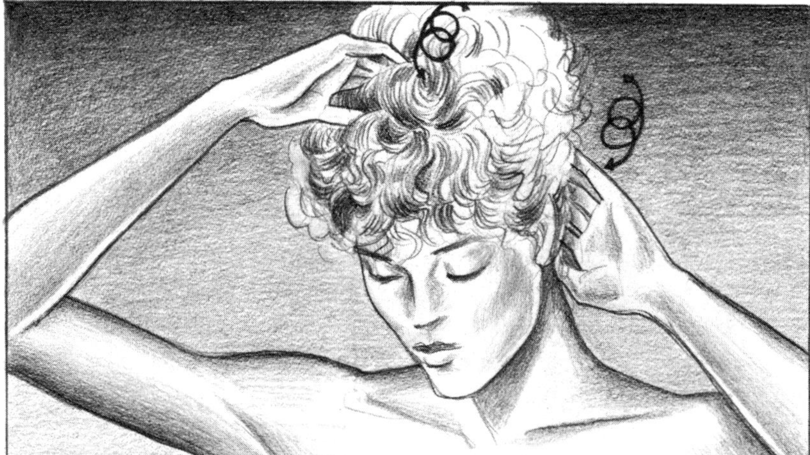

nape and hairline areas

hair a healthy shine. (If you have fine blond hair that's oily, use real, fresh lemon juice in the rinse and then rerinse with ice-cold water; brunettes or redheads can use 1 tablespoon of white vinegar.)

Use the old-fashioned squeak test to see if your hair is clean. If your hair doesn't squeak, rinse again.

To dry hair:

1. Towel-dry your hair to take out excess moisture. Press out the water by blotting.
2. Don't brush or comb your hair while wet. If you've washed by my method, you should have hardly any tangles or knots.
3. If you have the time, it is best to allow your hair to dry naturally. Style it while it is damp. Use a hair dryer only to shape the top, and let the fresh air dry the rest. If you have to use a dryer for the entire mane, don't use the hottest temperature, and keep the dryer at least nine inches away from your head to prevent burning and damaging hair and scalp. Use dryers as infrequently as possible. While there are conditioners to protect your hair from dryer damage, they tend to make the hair oily and kill the natural shine, so I don't recommend them.

Choosing shampoo, conditioners and rinses:

1. Remember, your scalp can be oily and your hair can be dry, so pick the products you use carefully. (It's impossible for your scalp to be dry and your hair to be oily, though!)
2. The finest hair is usually the oiliest, because there are more hairs and therefore more oil glands.
3. Choose your shampoo for its ability to control your scalp problems, then condition the hair accordingly.
4. Sun, hair color, perms, rollers (electric), blow dryers and swimming all can damage hair. Make sure you condition your hair accordingly.
5. Dry shampoos sound great for bad weather, travel or illness, but they never really clean the hair and scalp as well as regular shampoo.
6. If you have limp or flyaway hair, use the yolk of an egg to condition your hair. This gives fullness by separating the hairs. Be sure to rinse well in cool water. Hot water will cook the egg!
7. If you have dark hair, rinse with ½ cup of white-wine vinegar mixed with a quart of water to give your hair greater shine.
8. If you have blond or dirty-blond hair, rinse with camomile tea (1 cup loose tea leaves, strained with ½ quart water; leave on for 20 minutes) for greater shine and slightly lighter color.
9. Don't ever believe that all shampoos are created equal. They may be equally good cleaning agents, but what they do to your scalp and hair depends on your body condition and chemistry. So beware, and choose carefully! There are new shampoos for oily hair that are not too harsh. Read the labels and experiment with small sizes of new products.
10. If you have fragile hair, look for the chemical cyclometicine in your conditioner—it will help keep hair from breaking after shampooing.
11. Switching brands of shampoo is excellent, once you find the right types for your hair and scalp. Clear shampoos are usually stronger; creamy shampoos have some conditioner added. Many hair professionals recommend that you rotate brands. I find hair gets used to a shampoo quickly, so alternate brands every week or with every other shampooing. (It's also good to have a slightly milder shampoo and a slightly stronger one for different seasons—summer calls for a stronger shampoo if you've been perspiring a lot.)
12. Protein-enriched conditioners usually

add thickness to hair, giving you a little boost of body.

13. If a conditioner says you leave it on your hair, leave that brand on the shelf.

A DICTIONARY OF HAIR-PRODUCT BUZZWORDS

With competition for your dollar so keen, each manufacturer of shampoo and conditioner wants to convince you his product is the best. Hence glamour words, fancy chemicals and new ingredients are always being touted as the latest in beauty formulations. Here are some of my favorites:

Henna: Henna is a root that has been used to give reddish color to hair since ancient times. It also comes in a *natural* form that will add luster and body to hair without changing its color. If a product is marked "henna," check to see whether it is intended to highlight your hair or just to give it more body. There's no reason to end up a redhead by accident. (See page 75.)

Jojoba: Jojoba (pronounced "ho-HO-ba") is a plant that provides natural conditioning and is often added to shampoos or conditioning treatments.

Amino acid: Amino acids are a type of protein that gives your hair holding ability. They are available in shampoos and conditioners.

Placenta: The FDA discourages the use of placenta (usually cow placenta) in hair products because it is hard to rinse out. Pass.

Medicated: Medicated shampoos are usually for dandruff treatment and include a variety of chemicals that may or may not reduce flakiness. Remember that many cases of flakiness are not dandruff, so a dandruff treatment will sometimes not prove helpful. There are also nonmedicated dandruff shampoos—they contain fewer chemicals. Before choosing a "medicated" shampoo, get some professional advice on your scalp condition. There are no "medicated" conditioners.

PERSONAL HAIR POLICIES

No matter who cuts or styles your hair, or how happy you are with a salon, your hair will not look its best if you don't care for it properly. Shine doesn't come from a bottle or a layered cut—it comes from *within*!

■ Hair, like skin, has types. Learn which type you have and what it can and can't do. Your hair will be either curly, wavy or straight; fine, coarse or average in texture; thin, thick or average in quantity. While chemical treatments can alter some of these variables, it's always easiest if you can find a style that works with what it does best naturally. If you have curly hair, it's better to love it than to keep straightening it. Everyone, it seems, covets another kind of hair. My hair is straight and I always wanted curly hair. Jacquie's hair is curly and she's wanted straight hair—so badly she's even taken to ironing her curls. You just can't seem to win. But try to like what God gave you. You'll be a happier person and you'll save time and money.

■ Have the ends of your hair trimmed every two to three months if you have long straight hair. If you have a short style, you probably have your hair cut every six to eight weeks to keep the shape. If you just need your bangs trimmed or shaped, this can be done less expensively.

■ A good hairbrush with a rubber bed and natural bristles is worth the investment. The rubber bed eliminates static electricity, and the gentle, flexible bristles will last a long time. Mason Pearson is one of the best on the market.

■ Don't hide behind your hair. When you're younger and don't have the self-confidence you will develop later, you may find it easy to take cover behind bushy bangs and yards of hair. This is bad—both for your skin and for your psyche.

■ A certain amount of hair loss from brushing or shampooing is normal; don't worry about it. But if your hair is coming out in handfuls, see a doctor. Remember, medical treatments can make your hair fall out. Pregnancy and birth-control pills may cause an increase in the level of hair loss as well.

■ Never use an ordinary rubber band; use the covered kind, or a ribbon or large clips, to control your hair.

■ Keep all your hair-care tools clean. Once a week wash brush and combs in soapy water and then alcohol (Be sure to rinse well) or Barbicide (a disinfectant you can buy in a beauty-supply store), which should be diluted to a pale blue and then rinsed off with water.

■ Don't lend and don't borrow hair tools.

■ Only use a wide-tooth comb. A comb with teeth that are close together will break your hair.

■ Avoid hair spray. It coats your hair and attracts dust and dirt. Particles from the mist remain in the hair and may fall on your skin causing it to break out. Spray can have a drying effect on your hair . . . and your skin. No matter how "new" or "improved" the product—forget it.

■ Don't keep an electric roller in your hair longer than three minutes. Use wrapping papers on the ends of your hair whenever possible. It's best to heat the rollers, unplug them and then use them, so that they are never at their hottest.

HAIR APPLIANCES AND DOODADS

Each Christmas, new hair appliances come on the market as gift items. Some are new versions of the same old thing; others are totally new gadgets you never thought you needed until you saw the ad in a magazine.

Hair dryers: For the past ten or fifteen years, hand-held hair dryers have been the most important hairstyling appliance for men and women. You can still buy the old-fashioned hood dryer, and you can also buy a hood-and-hose attachment for your blow dryer. Hoods are good in winter, when you might not want to walk around your home with damp hair. They are also convenient for roller and pin-curl dries, because they free your hands. Just don't stay under the hood too long or turn the heat up too high or you'll damage your locks.

If you are using a hand-held hair dryer, 1200 watts will sufficiently dry your hair. I find 1000 watts not quite peppy enough (but excellent if you have thin or fragile hair) and 1500 watts too strong. I use a hair dryer that can be converted to 110 or 220 volts, so that I can travel anywhere in the world and not need to worry about electricity problems.

Diffusers: Many hand-held hair dryers are sold with a plastic end piece called a diffuser. It forces the hot air into a wider pattern, so that you do not concentrate a hot blast in one area. The diffuser helps prevent hair damage but is cumbersome to use.

Curling irons: There are several different types on the market, but the basic principle is the same—you plug in the heating rod and apply it to isolated sections of your hair. I think curling irons are great when someone else (usually a professional stylist) uses them but are awkward for home use. I've tried a few times and have burned the side of my face. I also wish I were an octopus as I reach my arms around trying to get into the right position for each tendril.

Crimpers: An electric crimper is a flat curling iron that looks a bit like a waffle iron. A hunk of hair (smaller than a section, more than a few strands) is laid in its jaws, the two parts are clamped together for a few seconds and the hair is pressed into a pattern of grooves. The effect on your hair is much the same as if you had put a wet finger into an electrical socket. Crimping is another technique that is difficult to perform on yourself. I also think it's a fun fad and not for classic beauties.

Electric rollers: Electric rollers can be damaging to your hair, but some varieties are less harmful than others. Some are heated with steam; some are coated with Teflon—investigate carefully. Any kind of heat will hurt your hair, especially when used constantly.

Pipe cleaners: If you want a curly permed look without crimping or using electric rollers, you can use pipe cleaners on your hair. Rags were the original hair rollers; pipe cleaners work by the same principle but give you a smaller, tighter curl. Wrap the tip of a strand in the pipe cleaner, roll toward the scalp, then twist the ends to secure the curl. Let dry.

Slightly more expensive, but somewhat easier to manage are the new flexible rollers that function much as the pipe cleaners do but will give you a looser, softer wave.

HAIR PROBLEMS

Hair treatments vary from deep conditioners you can use yourself to pills and injections you think will improve the shine or body of your hair. Many work; many do not.

If you are interested in a treatment to make your hair *thicker,* forget it. You're wasting time and money. Even a medical doctor cannot help you. Hormones may make your hair coarser—but not thicker. Conditioners only coat the hair to make it seem thicker.

Anesthesia administered before surgery may cause dramatic hair loss. No need to worry, unless the problem persists beyond six months: it may sometimes take that long for all the medication to work its way out of your body. This happened to a friend of mine who had gone in for a nose job. After all was said and done, she loved her new nose, but became deeply depressed because her hair was falling out by the handful. She went to several dermatologists, who did no more than prescribe lotions and potions. She spent a great deal of time and money, until, finally, one doctor asked her if she'd had any surgery recently and reassured her that time would remedy the situation. Although this problem doesn't affect everyone who has had surgery, it can happen.

Lice is a rare but not unheard-of problem. If you have terrible itching on the scalp, examine your hair and scalp under bright light. (If it's difficult to see into your hair, cut off about six strands and take a good hard look.) Should you see white specks on your hair (not your scalp) that resemble dandruff but that move when you use a magnifying glass, run to your dermatologist. He or she will treat the lice with a special shampoo that will kill them on contact. You must tell your parents, lovers, friends, family and everyone else with whom you've had close personal contact about this highly contagious problem. All clothes and bed linens must be laundered immediately, and linens should be changed daily until the problem is cured. All host environments must be destroyed. Don't forget to disinfect your hairbrushes, combs and makeup brushes.

SCALP AND DANDRUFF PROBLEMS

Some hair problems are treated with special scalp masks and ointments which are then beneficial to the hair. A scalp massage and steaming may or may not help you, depending on your problem. Scalp-massaging treatments are usually available at salons and are much like facials except that they are for the skin on *top* of your head. Such a treatment helps clean the scalp, helps cure dandruff and itchiness and can relieve oiliness . . . it's also infinitely relaxing. Massaging the scalp does not make your hair grow faster, better, stronger or fuller because the hair roots are stimulated and healthy due to blood flow. It *does* keep the hair roots healthy by bringing more blood to the surface. Remember, the perfect healthy scalp is not shiny, not flaky, not broken out, not tight, not itchy and not bumpy. It is clean and comfortable. Because we cannot see our own scalps it's always beneficial to have a professional look to see if you need treatment.

I had a client once who complained to me about dandruff and turned out to have a sunburned scalp. The tender skin on your scalp does indeed burn and peel just like the rest of your body. A hat will solve this problem.

If you actually do have dandruff, have a professional check it out and make a suggestion. There are many new coal-tar products available (The terrible aroma has been eliminated!), and no, coal tar has not been found to cause cancer—the Mayo Clinic has just finished a twenty-five-year study and found no increased risk. It's possible that dandruff is related to hormone changes in the body, because it usually shows up in teenagers, not children. Severe dandruff is thought to be hereditary; stress and weather also contribute to those falling flakes. (Dandruff is more common in winter.) Sometimes the dandruff treatment is causing the flakiness, so professional guidance is the best revenge.

CHOOSING A HAIRCUT AND A HAIRSTYLIST

I always find choosing a hairstyle and stylist a very emotional experience. You approach the situation pre-programmed—you've seen magazines, books and movies that affect your opinion of what's fashionable, new and chic. You are attracted to certain looks either because they are "in," because you wish you could wear them or because of some fantasy you have about how you can (and may) look. You think you can telegraph a message to the world about how you feel about yourself and who you really are through a hairstyle; then you worry that you won't be able to re-create the hairstyle as well as the stylist does. (I never can!)

On top of all that, your mother has spent most of your life picking your hairstyles for you and inputting into your mental computer what *she* thinks looks good (and appropriate) on you. Especially in your teen years, it's hard to ignore your mother's opinion.

When Marie was nineteen and a college sophomore, invited to her first grown-up ball, she went to her mother's hairstylist for a gala coiffure. Her mother did not go with her—after all, Marie was not a child—but did pay for the cut and set. When Marie emerged, some three hours later, she was thrilled with her new look. The stylist had adapted the latest fashion look to Marie's oval face and given her a toss of curls across the crown of her head with layers of waves cascading beneath. Marie was overjoyed. Her mother was appalled. "I paid for that rat's nest and I will not have you looking like a hooker. Now you call the salon and have them wash that out and start all over!" Mom completely deflated Marie's excitement. In a pitched battle, Marie stood her ground. She paid her mother for the wash and set and tried to hold her curly head up as she danced all night.

Whether Marie looked good or bad, her point was well taken. Mothers have a habit of "ruining" their daughters' fantasies and hairstyles (especially hairstyles for special occasions) because they hate to see their little girls grow up, or they have rigid preconceptions of what they should look like. As a result, choosing a hairstyle becomes not a treat but a trauma.

I once went to a well-known Beverly Hills salon and asked to have my hair put up for a special occasion. The poor hairdresser was unable to do it. He tried and tried, but he just never got it right. I emerged from the salon a nervous wreck and $30 poorer. It had never occurred to me that some stylists *can't* do what you want. For special occasions, you need to have a trial run or to do a lot of careful research *before* the big date.

Most young women go to their mother's hairstylist until they have the financial means to choose their own. This might happen when they are away at college; but most college girls prefer to have their hair cut when they are on vacation because of the security—and approval—that goes with Old Faithful. College girls are more likely to experiment on their own with hair coloring than with hairstyles.

When you do decide on a new style, keep these factors in mind:

■ The type of hair you have. No matter how you crave a certain style, if your hair type isn't appropriate, you're heading for heartache.

■ Your lifestyle—can you perform the necessary upkeep, or is this yet another style only the hairdresser can make look really good?

■ Will the change of hairstyle mean a change in drying procedure? What will it look like if you don't dry it that way?

Are there other ramifications? Do you have *time* for this style? Will you need a perm for proper upkeep? Is your hair colored? The time to ask these questions is *before* the scissors start snipping away.

Never be afraid to change salons, or change stylists within a shop. Each salon has its own "look," and you may want something entirely different from what a particular salon can provide. Not all stylists are versatile. While many are good at creating one or two types of styles, whether because of limited ability or their own personal preference, their trademarks may not be right for you.

In Choosing a Stylist

1. Word of mouth is one of the best methods of discovering the right stylist. Don't be afraid to go up to a stranger and say, "I love your hair. Who cut it?"

2. Blindly approaching a stylist you have not researched is dangerous.

3. A good cut is always a worthwhile investment; no amount of curling and styling will cover up a second-rate cut. Get the best you can afford. If finances are a real problem, ask your favorite salon if it needs models, or call a beauty school and find out if it has a night when the students give free haircuts. (It's possible to get a free haircut at the fanciest salons in the world this way.)

Caryn was a senior in high school and felt left out of all the excitement when her friends looked through glossy magazines and talked about their fashion plans for college. Her mother still insisted that she wear her hair long, straight and off her face and not "rush things" by trying to look too sophisticated. She was approached at a shopping mall one weekend by a student at a local beauty school who needed to practice short haircuts and was looking for a model with long, straight but thick hair. Since the cut was going to be free, and Caryn had wanted a fashion cut, she eagerly agreed. She emerged from her freebie with a layered short cut that gave fullness and bounce to her hair and enlivened her whole face. Suddenly she was transformed from a gawky teenager with a pretty but plain face into a beautiful, eye-catching young woman. Her mom loved the new cut, and Caryn took a big emotional step forward as she grew from little girl toward woman with newfound confidence. Then her mom volunteered to be experimented on too!

4. Discuss your intentions with your stylist-to-be. If you say cut one inch, and he or she cuts more—never return. The stylist *must* honor your requests. He may express a contrary opinion—that's his point of view and he's entitled to it—but he should not ignore your wishes. After all, you are paying for a service. Be sure your demands are feasible, though.

5. If you don't like your hair, say so immediately. Most people are too intimidated to speak up. This is nonsense. Make what you want clear and then tell the stylist where he has and hasn't pleased you. Act firm and know your own mind; if you are wishy-washy, you will be treated accordingly. If the new style or cut is so bad that all you want to do is go home and wash it out, make your displeasure known immediately to the stylist or the salon manager—you shouldn't have to pay for a style that is poorly done or not what you asked for in the first place.

Salon Procedures

After you've chosen a salon, book an appointment. Few salons like street traffic.

■ If you have questions about procedure, ask the receptionist.

■ Wear pants or a skirt rather than a dress, because you will be putting on a smock in the changing room and most smocks are not long enough to cover more than your fanny. Wear a buttoned top so you don't have to pull a sweater over your new hairstyle.

■ Dress carefully. Put on your makeup properly. Your grooming, your jewelry, your shoes and bag are all clues to stylist and staff that you are serious about what you look like.

■ Check in with the receptionist when you arrive. Go to the changing room and put on a clean smock.

■ When you emerge, catch the receptionist's eye and she will tell you where to wait or who will be shampooing your hair. If the shampooist asks if you want conditioner, remember to ask if you will be charged for it. Don't be afraid to say no.

■ If you are offered tea, coffee or wine, there will be no cost to you. (If you send out for lunch, you are expected to pay for the lunch and tip the person who brings it to you.) You do not have to tip the person who brings you the coffee or tea.

■ When your hair is finished, return to the dressing room to change into your street clothes. Then go to the receptionist to pay your bill. After paying, tip the various people involved in making you beautiful: tip 15 percent of the total bill to the stylist and 5 percent to the shampoo person. *Do not* tip the salon owner. If you see him being tipped by other people, ask the receptionist if the owner accepts tips; she will guide you.

■ If you go regularly to a salon, a small Christmas present may be in order. Usually, the staff prefers cash, or a heavy tip for extra work, special occasions or Christmas. If your regular appointments are with the owner, whom you have not been tipping, a bottle of wine or a thoughtful present would be appropriate.

■ If you cannot remember what the shampoo person looks like, ask the receptionist who shampooed your hair. The receptionist keeps envelopes for tips. Be sure to write *"Thank you! Stefi Fein"* on the envelope or something that tells the person who you are. Don't forget to tip the coat-check girl or the attendant in the dressing room (50 cents) if there is one.

■ If you have no money for a tip, say something about it to the stylist. "I'm low on cash this week; I'll get you next time" or something to explain your situation. If you plain old can't afford to tip, ask if you can make it up some other way—baby-sitting services, typing and so on—when you feel this would be appropriate.

Watch Out For:

■ A state license. It should be visible. If no license is in plain sight, take your business elsewhere.

■ Long waits. If you have waited for more than twenty minutes, leave. And tell the receptionist why. (If your hair has already been shampooed and you can't wait, ask for a dryer so you can blow it dry yourself. Do not pay for the shampoo or tip anyone.) It's not a bad idea to call the salon before you leave home to see if your stylist is on schedule. Often a regular is late and is given preference over you, or you may be given short shrift because you are younger. I think that anyone who keeps you waiting twenty minutes owes you an apology!

FINANCIAL NOTES

If finances are a consideration (aren't they always?), remember these things:

■ In big cities, most salons have an expert who does special work for major occasions and who is used infrequently by his or her clients. This person's specialty might be French braiding, weaving flowers into the hair or some other technique he may be able to teach you how to do.

■ Most salons will comb out your hair for you, which is less expensive than a wash and dry or wash and set. You wash your hair at home, dry it and use the electric rollers or your usual curling technique. The stylist just does the comb-out. Less cost, but a benefit from professional hands.

■ Salons charge for conditioner. If you are trying to save money, ask the shampoo person not to add conditioner. Often the pressure is intense ("But honey, your hair really *needs* it") and you end up paying $3–10 for a treatment when you could have bought a whole tube of the product for the same price. Just be firm.

PERMANENTS

In the last ten years, permanents have become highly fashionable on the American beauty scene. As a result, dozens of new formulas have been invented; there are permanents for people with fragile hair, colored hair, people who don't want curl but do want body, and many other variations as well. You can have a perm on the ends or at the scalp; you can have a perm on rods or big rollers. You name it and it's probably just been developed or is on the drawing board. So if your hair simply hangs there when you want it to bounce, consider a perm. If you want movement and texture and body, there's probably a method for you. But in exchange for your newfound fullness and easy care, don't forget you will be losing a lot of natural shine. And no matter how carefully the perm is given, it's still chemical and will never be a blessing to your hair. No chemical can be.

First of all, two definitions.

Body wave—a body wave is a perm timed for a short fix and used to put supplementary body into your hair without causing a frizzy or curly look.

Permanent—a perm is a chemical treatment that, depending on strength, formulation and how it's applied, can make your hair do anything but tap-dance.

The main idea behind the recent perm craze, other than to make you look like Little Orphan Annie, is to give you an easy-to-manage look. Permed hair can often dry naturally, which saves time, saves you from blow-drying damage and saves you from the age-old embarrassment of just not being able to do your hair as well as the stylist. If you are pregnant, if your hair has been colored or if you've recently had a perm, you should be especially careful about adding more chemicals to your hair.

Whatever you do, *don't* give yourself a perm, and do get good, solid professional advice.

Lara was a young working woman for whom things were going awry. She had just broken up with her boyfriend, was concerned about keeping her job, had blown her savings on a trip to Bermuda with her now ex-boyfriend and felt really fragile and unsure of herself. To brighten up her life, she decided to give herself a home perm (all she could afford). When the perm backfired and she ended up with patchy curls and marcelled waves rather than cascading curls, she panicked. She felt compelled to call in sick—further jeopardizing her position. Then she had to go to one of the best salons in town (borrowing $$$ from a friend) to have her hair cut very short and re-permed so she would look acceptable in the real world.

The moral of the story: perms can be tricky, and no matter how easy the box says it is, don't do it yourself. (If you insist on the home method, have a friend or family member apply the perm. Do NOT give yourself a perm if you have any real respect for your hair! And never do anything to your hair because you are depressed.) Permanents have come a long way, and disasters are rarer than before, but they are not foolproof.

If you are considering a perm:

- Go to a pro. (Please.) Preferably one who already knows your hair.
- Know the difference between a body wave and a permanent and see if the body wave will go the distance for you. Body waves are usually kinder to hair and scalp because they are not as strong or are given on larger-sized rollers and left on for a shorter time period.
- Do not have more than one perm a year.
- Do not back-to-back a perm with a hair-color treatment.
- Do not get a perm if you have sores, skin irritations or open scratches on your scalp.
- Make sure your stylist does a test curl before the perm is scheduled.
- Respect the strength of chemicals. Permed hair *must* be conditioned. Be sure you are willing to take the time to take care of your hair.
- If you are having an attack of the uglies (Don't laugh—everyone has them), don't go out and get a perm because you think it will make your life better. It will take months to grow out completely (unless your hair is very short), so think about this step seriously.
- Getting a permanent reduces the hair's natural shine—it's a trade-off.

HAIR COLORING

Hair coloring has ancient roots, if you'll excuse the pun, and has long been considered an exciting way to brighten up your appearance—and often help the condition of your hair. (The addition of color or rinse coats the hair, making it seem thicker, and thus gives a little more body to limp hair.) Because there are now so many different hair-coloring techniques, products and tricks, I thought we should start with a mini-dictionary.

Permanent hair color: Stays on the hair shaft and grows out at the speed at which your hair grows, so that your natural color re-emerges at the roots within three to six weeks. It requires constant upkeep to cover the new growth. I recommend this process only for covering gray hair. There are other ways to add zest to your hair color that don't lead to root problems.

Semi-permanent hair color: Washes away a little bit each time you shampoo; expect it to last three to six washings. Great for beginners!

Rinse: A type of semi-permanent hair color. It usually lasts one week, or until the next washing. Good for parties or impulse coloring because it will not last and you won't have to live with a mistake.

Frosting: Process by which strands of hair are pulled through holes in a cap and are then lightened, after which the entire head is treated with a toner. This provides various shades of blond to lighten up an otherwise mousy-brown head of hair.

Weaving: Hair is sectioned; then the tail of a comb is used to weave through and select a few hairs for coloring. This way the color is subtle and well distributed, actually woven into your natural shade. A good technique when your hair is beginning to turn gray and you don't want the drudgery of permanent hair color.

Hair painting: (also called *balayage,* pronounced "bah-lay-AHZH"). Lightener is painted on various strands of hair to give casual, random highlights. There is no pattern to the painting, so regrowth is not apparent. You can retouch every three to four months. If you are interested in home coloring, hair painting is a simple method that is almost fail-safe.

Half-head coloring: Most streaking processes can be done on just the crown of the head and made to blend with your natural color. This is less expensive than if you have the entire head streaked. Often women like to alternate between the whole head and the half head, every three to four months.

Stripping: The natural hair color is removed with chemicals and then a new (and different) hair color is applied. If you desire a much lighter color, your hair will have to be stripped first. This bleaching/stripping combo is known as two-process coloring.

Henna: Pure henna is a mash made of henna leaves that will redden hair—the intensity is, of course, dependent on your natural color. (It hardly even shows up on black hair.) There is also compound henna, in which henna leaves are combined with chemicals for different color possibilities—but those chemicals are usually very harsh on the hair. Beware of discoloration and hair damage. Neutral henna will not give you any color at all and is excellent for adding body.

DO-IT-YOURSELF COLOR

For as many types of hair-coloring methods as now exist, there are as many kits and do-it-yourself procedures that tell you how to achieve the look you want by yourself or with a friend's help. Two-process hair-color jobs are difficult and take a chemist's hand, and frosting is difficult to perform (you have to pull the hair through a cap with a crochet hook), but many other types of hair coloring are fun and easy to experiment with at home.

Because helping Mother Nature make your hair color a little more special is no longer considered cheating, young girls are often allowed to experiment. When I was little, my mother used a camomile tea rinse on my hair. Evan was seven when her stepmother started to lighten her hair. Evan's hair was the kind of dirty-blond–mousy-brown that automatically got lighter in the summer, so her stepmother just accelerated things. The summer Evan was seven, her stepmom mixed a brew of lemon juice and vinegar. The next summer, she began using a hair-painting kit she bought at the dime store to give Evan a little more sunshine than was really coming her way. Now fifteen, Evan uses a summer lightener that she applies herself three times a year.

When I was in college, a lot of the girls liked to use a lightening shampoo by Roux that helped keep their hair a little more blond or red (as the case was) than it naturally was. There was one girl who decided to become a redhead and had disastrous results with peroxide. Another tried a summer-sun product that she sprayed on, then went out in the sun, only to return with orange hair—probably because the bottle wasn't fresh.

Because all hair-coloring products involve chemicals, they should be treated with caution and concern. Always use extra care not to get lotions in your eyes, and be sure to wear rubber gloves. (A ring with prongs can tear through the gloves, so remove jewelry before you put on the gloves.)

■ If possible, have a *consultation* with a professional colorist, even if you plan to do the color yourself. You may well have the colorist do it the first time, then teach you how to do the upkeep. This is usually worth the initial investment. (Tip the colorist 15 percent of the color bill, which will vary with each procedure, but you can guess it will be between $25 and $150. Ask first.)

■ NEVER use peroxide out of the bottle on your hair.

■ Avoid products that ask you to use sunshine to help them develop—the sun is no better for your hair than it is for your skin, and you have no control over the effects of the rays. The color you get may come as a big surprise.

■ Color can never give hair a better shine. In fact, it actually strips the natural oils that give hair its healthy shine. Artificial color may supply more light, but it will never replace the healthy shine natural hair has when it's been well taken care of. Samantha had the shade of dirty-blond hair that leads all women who have it eventually to begin lightening their hair. While she should have stayed with streaks, she went instead to permanent hair color. As years passed and the damage continued, she kept making the color more blond to compensate for the fact that she was steadily dimming her natural shine. Now it's plain old brassy.

■ Streaks are always better than overall color, since the untouched hair will have natural shine. When you style your hair, the combination is very effective.

■ Avoid fad hair-color trends. (See page 77.)

■ If you are coloring your hair for fun (rather than to cover gray), choose streaking, hair painting or hair weaving; you should resort to overall permanent color only when you are covering gray. There is no need to be a slave to your roots before you are forty.

In choosing your new hair color, match to your skin tones; but remember that as you age, natural color changes, usually growing a bit darker. So if you color your hair, coordinate it with your skin tone *and* your original hair shade, or make it a little bit lighter. Making your hair darker will make you look *older*.

■ If you decide to let your hair grow back to its natural color, get some professional help. It may take a full two years to restore your natural shade, so be patient.

We had a very attractive client, named Renée, who had come to us for a makeup consultation. Usually, when I look at someone, I instinctively know which colors of foundation, eye shadow and lip tones to use. But with Renée, I just couldn't decide. Nothing seemed right. She had light olive skin, greenish-brown eyes, dark eyebrows—and very blond hair. After mentally going through six different color combinations, I finally realized just what the problem was. Renée wasn't *meant* to be a towhead. Her coloring was for ash-blond to pale brown hair. No matter which makeup I selected, it was going to be wrong either for the skin or for the hair color. Blond tones wouldn't work with her skin, and olive wouldn't work with her hair! If you plan to fool Mother Nature, you have to be tactful.

You can always try the old department-store wig trick, if you are thinking of a change, but the best changes are subtle ones that make your hair appear livelier, not different. Go a shade lighter or a shade darker in the beginning, no more. Do not try permanent hair color as an experiment, because it's unlikely you will be able to match it back to your natural shade. Your skin tone, eye color and even wardrobe should be guides when you pick a new hair color.

When Tara went away to college, she couldn't wait—finally out of range of her mother's watchful gaze—to turn her dark brown hair the auburn she had always wanted. Tara thought she looked divine as a redhead. Except that all her red and burgundy clothes—which had looked great with her dark brown hair—clashed with her new look. At first, Tara tried everything from more beauty sleep to more makeup. But finally, she was forced to surrender. Without funds to totally revamp her cosmetics and closet, Tara had to return to a medium brown shade until her own hair color could grow out.

Always have a strand test in a salon, or test yourself at home. Cut a small amount of hair from the back and apply color according to directions. You'll see the true color you'll be getting and avoid a lot of mistakes.

FAD HAIR COLOR

Just as fashion fads run in cycles, there are often hair-color fads. The platinum-blond look was "in" during the 1950s, henna became popular in the late 1960s and the '80s have fallen victim to the influences of punk rock-'n'-roll. Along with punk clothes, the punk hairstyle often demands that a section or strand of hair be stripped and recolored with a vegetable dye, so the wearer can have a dash of red, green, blue, turquoise or purple hair.

While something like this may be amusing, even appealing, it should not be done on a whim, because it's hard to re-color a section of hair to match the rest of your tresses. It will take six months to a year for the color to grow out unless you cut off your hair—so think about it a long time before you get involved in any fads.

The ideal color change restores hair to the shade it was in childhood. And I know you didn't have blue streaks then!

EYEBROW COLOR

While women may spend a lot of time and money to color their hair a new shade, they often neglect their eyebrows. Nothing is a bigger giveaway that you've been tinkering than a light head and dark brows . . . and nothing (unless you're Margaux Hemingway) looks tackier! If you aren't a natural, at least try to coordinate your hairy zones. (It was even fashionable in the glory days of Hollywood for celebrities to dye their pubic hair to match their hair and brows—that final convincing touch.)

Eyebrows should be one to two shades darker than hair for light hair and matching for dark hair. Bleaching brows yourself can be risky—you can end up with orange eyebrows. NEVER apply hair dye to your eyebrows; it can drip into your eyes too easily. There are special eyebrow formulas to use, if you are a do-it-yourselfer. I suggest, instead, that you go to a pro. It's better to have the brows come out too dark and need a reapplication of bleach than to go too light and hate yourself for months. Even if you don't have your hair colored at a salon, let a pro do your eyebrows, please.

WIGS AND OTHER HAIRPIECES

While wigs at the beauty shop and on actresses always look alluring, in real life they usually look artificial. There is only one time when you should wear a wig: when you don't have any hair.

Hairpieces are fun for special occasions, but they go into and out of style and are rarely worth the investment. Cheap hairpieces *never* match and *always* look cheap.

The only good thing I can say about wigs is that if you are considering a drastic haircolor change, you can go to a department store and try on a wig in the proposed new shade to see how it looks with your skin and wardrobe. This exercise can spare you a lot of grief.

UNWANTED HAIR

The most important thing to consider in the removal of unwanted hair is that there is no one perfect method. Various techniques are best suited to different areas of the body. Budget can also enter the picture.

There are a few things about hair removal and regrowth that you need to know before you begin to tackle the problem.

- If you have blond peach-fuzz body hair, don't do anything to it. I wouldn't even shave the legs, but if you insist, just go to the knee.
- Once you start a hair-removal program, you become a slave to it.
- Hair often grows back darker and coarser. (That's why blond peach fuzz should be left alone.)
- Depending on the area of the body, the hair-removal techniques are more or less sophisticated and remove only a percentage of the unwanted hairs.
- Some methods may be painful. Others may be painful *and* expensive. Get a good grounding in the various options before you pick one. Always consider professional help. Some hair-removal techniques should *not* be practiced by do-it-yourselfers. Check the box for exact information on each of the types of hair removal.

HAIR-REMOVAL TECHNIQUES

Shaving: Shaving is a great technique for under the arms and an adequate method for the legs. Since the hair is cut off at the surface, it grows in quickly—usually within a day or two. Since hair grows faster in summer than in winter, more frequent shavings are necessary then. Always use a sharp razor; never borrow someone else's razor (especially your man's), because it may be dull and nick you or you will dull it and the owner will be mad at you. Make sure your skin is wet and pliable when you shave; always use a lathering of soap or a shaving cream.

Depilatories: Creams and lotions that chemically dissolve the hair so that it falls off at either the skin's surface or the hair root (depends on type of product) have been on the market for many years. They used to be very smelly and cause rashes—now some have been improved. Always do a patch test first, to check for allergic reaction. Hair must be treated every seven to fourteen days. This method is best for legs.

Bleach: Bleach in a cream base is easy and safe to use, as long as you follow the instructions and keep careful track of the time. If the bleach is taken off too early, hairs will be a pale shade of orange; reapply until the hairs are see-through blond. If you leave bleach on too long, you may develop a rash or burn. If bleaching eyebrows, be sure to protect your eyes. Should any bleach get in your eyes, flush them with water immediately.

Wax: There are two types of wax methods for removing hair—hot wax, in which the wax is melted, painted on with a tongue depressor and removed cum hair, and cold wax, which is removed with linen or muslin strips. There are cold-wax kits for at-home use; hot wax should never be attempted at home. Although this method can be painful, it is an excellent technique because the hair is pulled up from the root, so it lasts the longest. The first session is always the most painful; after a few sessions, pain is minimal because less hair has grown in and you have become accustomed to it. Many people look like a plucked chicken after waxing, so don't plan to go directly to the beach. Redness may last overnight. If you are having a leg wax and have a cut or scab, be sure to let the person doing the work be aware of it. Don't assume she will automatically avoid it. Removing a scab prematurely might cause a scar, so be certain to inform the technician.

Electrolysis: A needle is inserted into each hair follicle, destroying the root with an electrical jolt. The results are permanent once all the hairs are removed, which may take several treatments. Can be painful. Use a qualified expert and investigate techniques. The needles can cause scarring if the insert is too deep, and the visit can be fruitless if it isn't deep enough. This is a difficult procedure.

Now let's go at this by parts of the body.

Legs

The most effective hair-removal method for the legs is waxing. It is also expensive and somewhat painful. The pain is really only momentary and is worst the first time. The leg is slathered with hot or cold wax. When the wax is lifted off, the underlying hair goes along with it. This feels a lot like removing a Band-Aid. The skill and speed of the operator is key. Waxing is a deep removal, so it lasts as long as six weeks, a little less for coarser hair.

Shaving your legs is the least expensive method, but increases the chance of self-inflicted wounds. Nicks hurt and are ugly—especially if you are not wearing stockings. Shaving breaks off the hair at the point where razor meets hair and does not get it out of the shaft the way waxing does. Shaved hair grows back quickly, so it's not uncommon for shavers to have to de-fuzz once a day—especially in summer or on winter vacation in tropical climes.

Cream removers, while effective, often cause irritations, rashes or itching. They leave skin smooth, but require patience. The cream must remain on the skin about fifteen to twenty minutes to be effective. Thus it is time-consuming and costly, and often smelly too. You can go longer between cream treatments than with shaving—but not nearly as long as with waxing. If you like the cream method, experiment with several brands—one may be kinder to your skin than another.

Crotch

The delicate term for hair removal around the pubis is "bikini hair removal." Popular within the last two decades, hair removal from this sensitive area is still something many women do not even know about. Depending on your hair type and growth pattern, you may have an embarrassing problem with pubic hair in your teen years, or you may never need to think twice. If, when you wear a swimsuit or leotard, you are worried that pubic hairs will peep out and embarrass you, you should consider one of several types of hair removal.

Never use a cream hair remover on this delicate area.

Never wax the pubic hair yourself. A bikini wax by a professional is probably the best way to remove unwanted pubic hair, but this should never be attempted at home. If you have a professional bikini wax, a towel is usually provided, and you wrap it around you like a diaper. However, I suggest wearing your favorite leotard or swimsuit if you are embarrassed. Whenever I think of home bikini waxing, I remember the story a fashion editor friend told me: A bride-to-be suddenly decided that she needed a bikini wax before her wedding. The wedding was scheduled at four in the afternoon on a Saturday—a very busy day for salons—and she could not get an appointment. She decided to do the job herself and ended up in the emergency room of her local hospital! If you ever consider waxing this area yourself, remember this poor bride!

Do not shave the pubic hair around the thighs, because it will grow back coarser and possibly denser. You can end up with a real beard! If you do not heed my advice and decide to shave pubic hair, do so carefully, and always shave up—not down. For a few stray hairs, use a tweezer; that way you can choose the hairs you wish to remove.

Remember, if you use a razor and inadvertently get some of the peach fuzz that is not pubic hair, it will grow back as coarse as pubic hair and you will have created a serious problem.

I've seen women on the beaches who have bleached their pubic hair. I do not recommend this, because when you are close, you still see the hairs. No matter how light your pubic hairs are, when they are peeping out of your swimsuit, they are not attractive.

Underarms

Shaving is an excellent technique for removing underarm hair. Creams need longish hair to grab on to, to be effective and can cause rashes, and waxing is painful because the underarm area is more sensitive than the legs. Shave every other day to give the hair enough of a chance to grow out so you are not shaving off skin. Always soak the underarm skin first, then apply a shaving cream to avoid irritation. In winter (when hair doesn't grow as fast) you can shave every two or three days.

Arms

If your outer arms are unnaturally hairy (with dark, not light, hair), bleach the hair. Do not shave it; wax if you must. Again, once you start using a razor, you will have to do it continually. Stubble looks awful after a few days. This is a procedure you can never go back on, so don't get carried away with a "brilliant idea" and suffer for years. After shaving, arm hair grows in aggressively to produce the famed gorilla effect.

Lips

Never shave the hair over your lips, even if you look like a boy. First try bleach. If that is unsuccessful, try waxing. There are hot and cold wax methods for this part of the body; cold wax is better for sensitive skin. Salons use both methods. Compresses should be applied after a hot wax. Electrolysis can solve the problem (although not necessarily permanently), but it's expensive and painful and could leave scars. It should be done in sections rather than all at once. Electrolysis is a very difficult procedure, which I know from doing it myself. You have to place the needle into the hair shaft down to the root and kill the hair. If you don't go far enough, the hair won't be dead and the process will be useless. If you go too far, the client will have a scar. What pressure! Because of the time involved in getting at each shaft, electrolysis is a costly and time-consuming process. And to top it off, hair grows in six-week cycles and some hairs are dormant, so you have to keep coming back for more treatments until all the hairs are killed. This is my least-favorite solution.

Breasts

Some women have a few hairs around their nipples. (The hair sometimes grows in as you age.) If the hairs do not bother you, or your boyfriend or husband, *ignore* them. If you are terribly self-conscious about them, bleach them. (You can do this yourself.) Never, never tweeze them, because your nightmare will come true—more hairs will grow in, and they will be as coarse as pubic hairs. If they are causing you dreadful anguish, investigate electrolysis. Your doctor should be able to recommend a good electrologist.

Five

Teeth and Mouth

THE MILLION-DOLLAR SMILE

It's true. Things *really* do go better when you smile. Your face lights up and the world lights up. Taking care of the components of your smile (and your kisses, for that matter) is an important investment not only in what you look like, but in how you act and feel.

Dental problems are no smiling matter, but unfortunately, they are so common that they are widely accepted as part of life. Few people realize that you can *fight* them and that you can *prevent* many so-called "common" problems before they happen. Nobody likes to go to the dentist, yet few do anything to obviate the experience or to make it a positive instead of a negative one.

Science has come a long way since George Washington wore his whalebone dentures, but no matter how sophisticated the fakes, nothing ever compensates for the originals. Real teeth are more comfortable, more natural-looking, more attractive, more supportive to face tissue and more capable of eating a variety of foods than anything else science has or will come up with. So make up your mind to take care of your mouth—inside and out—and your mouth will take care of you for a long, long time.

Smiling is a matter of style. If you think about it, there are many signature smiles identified with different people.

- The Miss America Smile—the big, toothy grin you see on young hopefuls who prance down beauty-contest runways. The professional politician practices a variant of this warm, open, confidence-inspiring grin.
- The Sly Grin—this shows either no teeth or perhaps two, usually the front top teeth, but experienced sly-grinners contrive to show you one top front tooth and the tooth next to it, rather than baring just the two biggies.
- One-Rowers—some people smile a full smile while managing to reveal only their top teeth. This is usually very sincere-looking without the forced look of the Miss America Smile. It's also excellent for people who don't have perfect teeth.
- The Cheshire Cat—this is achieved entirely with the face muscles and the eyes. No teeth show whatsoever.

Some smiles are hereditary; some smiles come naturally; some are practiced to perfection. But even a baby knows you win more friends with a smile than with a frown. Smiling is a social and political activity and has to be considered an important weapon in self-presentation. Some societies smile more than others; some peer groups smile more than others; some people encourage smiles; others discourage them.

To see the importance of a smile to your face and future, take the smile test. Go into one of those photo booths they have in dime stores, airports and subway stations, or get a friend with an instant camera to take several snapshots of you. Try a variety of smiles. Almost anyone should be able to come up with four different versions. An actress can probably do eight. Study your pictures carefully—note how various smiles change the contours of your face and project different messages. You may even want to pick the one you like best and practice it. Practice makes perfect, you know. (I always thought too much of my gums showed when I smiled, so I practiced holding my lip down until I got a smile I liked. An actress I know shared her secret with me: push your tongue to the front of the roof of your mouth, then smile.)

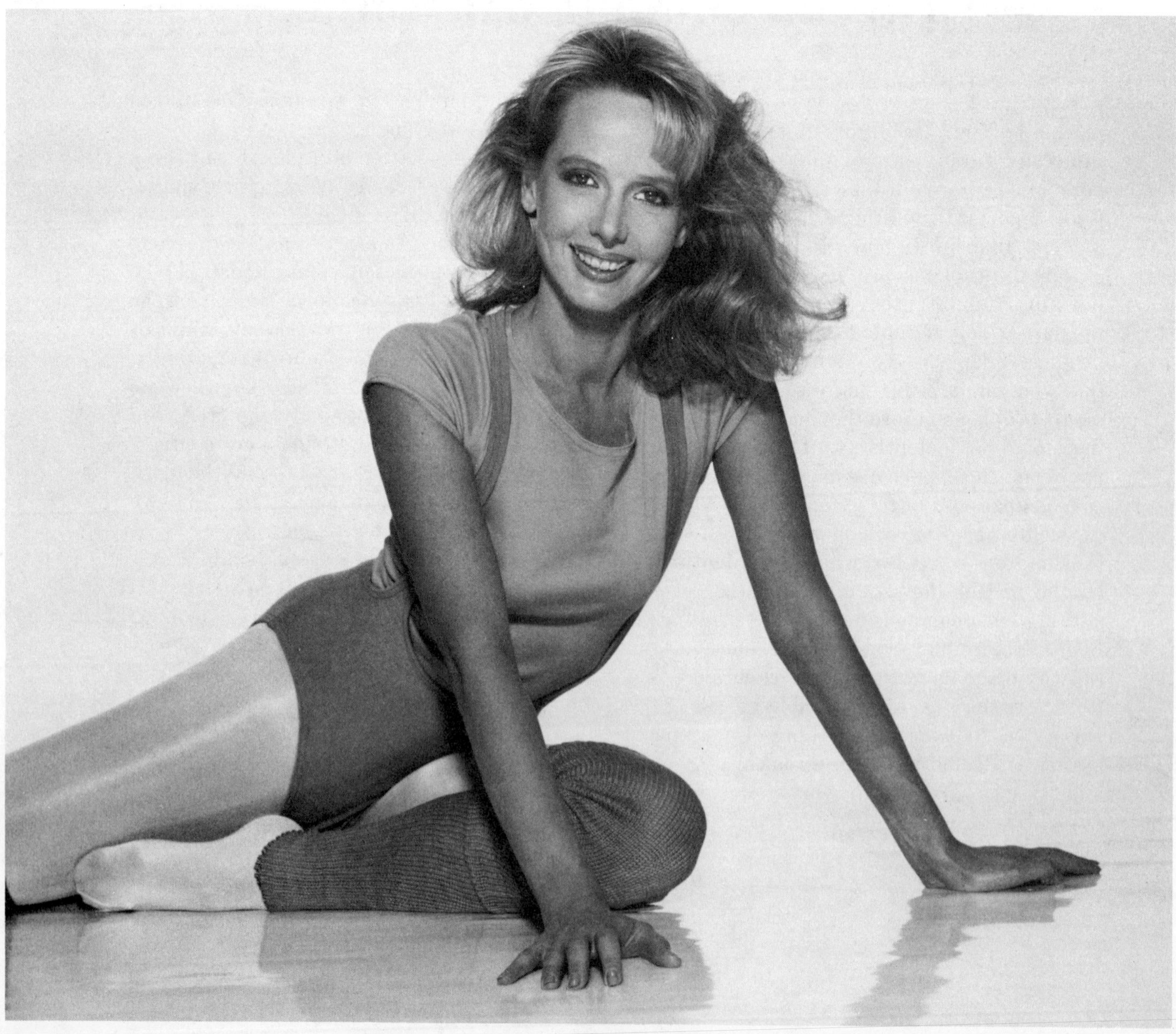

HEALTH AND HYGIENE

Behind every smile are the basics: teeth and gums. Some dental problems are inherited; most are man-made. A tremendous number are directly due to impaired personal health and inadequate hygiene.

■ Dental decay attacks 98 percent of the population.

■ By age two, 50 percent of the children in this country have tooth decay.

■ By age twenty, the average adult has decay in 14 of his 32 teeth.

■ Gum infection strikes 90 percent of the population.

■ Gum disease affects about three-quarters of the population before they are fifty years old.

■ One out of every ten people in this country has lost all his teeth.

■ Dental dysfunction is the world's third-most-common health problem.

So the next time you smile at yourself in the mirror, take another look. Are your teeth stained? Are they uneven? Do you look a bit like Dracula when you smile? Do you have dragon breath? Are there gaps in your mouth where there should be teeth? Is your smile all metal and glow? Many of these factors are within *your* control.

■ Teeth stain: there's no question about that. To keep them white, you need to protect them. Stay away from coffee, tea and cigarettes.

My friend Kim is a most attractive person until she smiles. Then she bares her badly yellowed teeth. Yet she still smokes two packs of cigarettes a day.

■ If it's not possible to brush your teeth between meals, at least rinse your mouth with water. This will help prevent acid buildup that attacks teeth and keep your breath a little sweeter, longer.

■ Think about what you are eating. Don't eat garlic-laden foods or Chinese, Mexican or other ethnic dishes known to be spicy before dates and interviews, if you work with others or in any situation in which you are concerned about your breath. Bad breath comes from the stomach, the teeth and the mouth. Protect all three by choosing what you eat carefully. If you just can't resist that garlicky bouillabaisse, be sure to carry a small bottle of mouth spray with you in your handbag, pocket or glove compartment. You never know whom you may run into. (I always keep a mouth spray in the glove compartment of my car and one in each handbag. No need to be embarrassed!)

■ Brushing is not enough to keep your teeth clean; you must floss every twenty-four hours.

■ See a hygienist every six months, at the very least, for a professional cleaning. This will help prevent cavities, gum disease and bad breath. It'll also save money, because a good hygienist will be able to spot trouble areas before they become disaster areas.

DENTAL DISEASE

There are two main forms of dental disease:

- tooth decay
- gum infection

You may have a problem in one area or the other, or a problem can start in one area and move on to infect the other.

Tooth decay is a fancy term for cavities, something you've been hearing about ever since you were old enough to begin watching TV. Tooth decay attacks the enamel and, if it is not caught in time, slowly corrodes the inside (dentin) of the tooth and can eat through to the nerve, which really hurts. You may not notice tooth decay before you feel the pain, which is one reason why regular checkups are crucial. The more the decay progresses, the more dramatic (and painful and expensive) the necessary treatment.

The main cause of tooth decay is *plaque,* a sticky film harboring bacteria that likes to adhere to the teeth and gums and the margin between them. The bacteria combine with the foods you eat—especially sugars—and produce an acid which attacks the enamel and sets the tooth-decay process into action. The best way to prevent cavities and tooth decay is through a regular program of personal and professional dental hygiene—and if you have a history of problems, you should see a dentist or hygienist three times a year.

Gum infection is also caused by plaque. The toxins produced by the bacteria in your mouth can lead to an inflammation that enlarges the space between the tooth and the gum. The plaque then collects in *this* space, causing an infection. The plaque hardens into tartar—a deposit that cannot be removed by brushing—and more plaque is collected, creating a vicious circle. If this condition is not treated, you get a gum disease called gingivitis. Slowly the supporting bone structure is eroded and destroyed until the tooth loosens and falls out. You probably cannot detect this ominous process yourself, so the help of an expert is imperative. Gum disease is rarely painful, but has these symptoms:

- tender gums that bleed when you brush your teeth
- swollen gums
- bad breath

BRUSHA BRUSHA BRUSHA

Brushing your teeth properly (and frequently) will make a big difference to their health, their proclivity toward cavity and decay, and the freshness of your breath.

Here are the supplies you'll need:

1. Not one, but two toothbrushes. One is

an adult toothbrush (Oral B is a good brand) with a soft and flexible nylon bristle. While there isn't one right type, do not buy hard-bristle brushes unless you need help cleaning your typewriter. The second toothbrush is child-size—great for getting to those back teeth which can't be reached by the larger brush!

2. Toothpaste. Toothpaste is largely a cosmetic, so choose by taste, color or packaging and texture. (Many dentists recommend you alternate two different fluoride pastes.) There are also toothpastes for sensitive teeth (Yes, some teeth are more sensitive than others) and tooth powders, which were used before pastes were invented and work just fine —only make sure yours is not abrasive.

3. Dental floss. Flossing is a must, no matter how time-consuming. Made of silk, cotton or nylon, floss may be either waxed or unwaxed, and is an essential tool for getting between the teeth where your brush can't possibly reach. The floss should be able to get in between each tooth and the next. If you need a flossing lesson, ask your hygienist. If floss doesn't fit between your teeth, see your dentist.

4. Disclosing tablets. These are made of red vegetable dye, and they stain the plaque so you can see exactly what you are and aren't getting clean when you brush your teeth. Don't worry: the stain is not permanent; brushing and rinsing will wash it away. These are great for showing children where they aren't brushing, but even adults should use them every now and then as a spot check. After all, being an adult doesn't necessarily mean you are brushing your teeth properly. (See page 88.)

5. Peroxide and baking soda. These are the key ingredients of a paste you make yourself for massaging your gums. Gum massage, also known as the Keyes Method, is a controversial technique for fighting decay. (Periodontists are not uniformly for it; most dentists are.) Every day you simply mix up a little paste of peroxide and baking soda (I pour it into my hand, using about a teaspoon of each) and work it around the teeth with the rubber tip on the end of your toothbrush. The formula is supposed to alter the acid balance in the mouth and therefore help kill the bacteria assaulting your gums. You can do the massaging with an electric toothbrush or a Proxabrush (a small brush you can buy at a drugstore). Dental floss also helps massage gums.

6. Other supplies. There are two new products you may want to consider as part of your mouth-cleaning ritual; one is a fluoride mouthwash and the other is an anti-plaque ingredient that you rinse with which is just getting FDA approval, so ask your dentist or hygienist about it. While I am not promoting brands, there are new products in the area of oral hygiene coming out every day.

Note: I have not put an ordinary mouthwash on this list because it is not essential in the cleaning of teeth and mouth and is primarily a cosmetic or psychological boost. While it may freshen your breath, it does not kill bacteria.

Toothpicks (the round, not the flat, ones) are excellent for *gently* scraping off plaque, especially right after meals. I've been doing it ever since my dentist recommended it to me. Be sure to reach those back teeth and do the front and back of each tooth.

HOW TO BRUSH

To brush properly, put the bristles of your regular-size (Use soft or medium, never hard bristles) brush at an angle to your teeth. Brush the top row downward—never brush horizontally; it's all in the wrist. Brush the bottom row upward. After brushing the front and back of the upper and lower teeth, use a child's brush for the hard-to-reach back teeth. Alternate sides when you begin to brush, because you will put more energy into brushing when you start out.

Buy new sets of toothbrushes every ten to twelve weeks.

FLUORIDE

One of the easiest ways to prevent cavities—and tooth decay—is to fight back with fluoride. Fluoride is available from several sources. Your local water supply may be fluoridated, you can buy toothpaste with fluoride in it and you can gargle with the new fluoride rinses. Up to two-thirds of all dental decay can be prevented by fluoride! (A recent study showed that fluoridation in the water reduces the eventual need for dentures by 30 percent.)

Fluoride protects the teeth by forming a protective layer of hydroxyapatite over the tooth enamel. This is a mineral coating that actually resists the acid created by bacteria.

According to most dental experts, fluoride in the water is safe and causes no known side effects. Even if you drink fluoridated water, brush with fluoridated toothpaste and use a fluoride rinse, you do not run a health risk. It takes eight times the dose in water just to cause teeth to discolor, so you are perfectly safe with the three types of treatments.

BAD MOUTHING

The teeth fit into your jaw and your jaw holds up your face, much like the foundation of a building, so your mouth is important not only in eating and kissing, but in keeping your features where they should be. (People with severe dental problems often look older because a change in their dentition causes the skin to droop.) Bad habits can affect your teeth, your gums and your face structure, so avoid:

- sucking your thumb
- biting your nails
- pushing your tongue up against your front teeth
- biting your cheeks (from the inside)
- chewing on your lips
- resting your chin or jaw on your fist
- sucking your lips, or any other nervous manifestation
- grinding your teeth
- clenching your jaw

BAD BREATH

Bad breath is a dread embarrassment because you seldom know you have it, while the people who have to deal with you may be secretly offended by it. It's a rare and valuable friend or associate who will mention that you have bad breath, yet it's a serious social problem that can drive people away.

Bad breath is caused by the foods you eat (particles becoming trapped between your teeth), the way your body digests and the state of your teeth and gums. Infection breeds odors. To keep bad breath to a minimum:

- Remember your semi-annual cleaning. If you have a problem with bad breath, four times a year is advisable.
- Brush your teeth after meals. Carry a portable toothbrush.
- Floss after meals.
- Avoid sugary foods—they cause decay and attract the bacteria that cause odor. If you can't brush your teeth after drinking a soda, skip it.
- Avoid offensive foods—onions, garlic, you know the list.
- Breath mints, sprays and mouthwashes may make you feel more confident, but they do not actually prevent or combat bad breath. Solve the problem; don't try to mask it.
- Investigate a product called a "Rush Brush"—it's a mint-tasting knit tube that fits on your finger and, when you can't brush, helps rub off breath offenders. No need to rinse. This is, however, no substitute for brushing or flossing.

DOCTOR TOOTH

There are several specialists who can help you in your fight against tooth and mouth disease. One, of course, is your dentist. But you should also know the full range of work other people in this field do, so you can pick the right specialists for your needs—needs that will vary at different stages of your life.

The dentist: The dentist is the overall caretaker of your mouth, whose main job is the analysis, care, cleaning and maintenance of your teeth and gums. If your problems require other action, he can refer you to a specialist, such as an oral surgeon or an orthodontist.

The dental hygienist: A hygienist may or may not work for or with a dentist and may be seen at the same time or separately. It's the hygienist who cleans your teeth professionally and checks for early warning signs of trouble. She can detect leaks in existing fillings as well as find new cavities. The hygienist can give you a more thorough cleaning than you can give yourself.

The periodontist: This specialization is up-and-coming. The periodontist is primarily interested in your gums, and the removal of plaque from the margin between your teeth and gums.

The orthodontist: A specialist in straightening and rearranging teeth.

The tooth fairy: Not related to any of the above.

Don't choose a dentist because you're chicken and he's nice. He must be qualified and do thorough work. I once had a dentist who was so nice, he was afraid to hurt me. So when I needed a cavity drilled out, he stopped too soon; not all the decay was removed, and I ended up having to have the entire process redone later on, and it hurt twice as much as the first time.

BRACES AND RETAINERS

As you begin puberty and your body settles into the shape it will have as an adult, you and your dentist may see the need for braces, a retainer or other orthodontic work. Some factors in tooth and jaw structure are hereditary (a space between your two front teeth is usually inherited!), so often the need for orthodontia is a family trait—one over which you have no control. After all, the basic challenge of orthodontia is to alter the structure of the bones that support your teeth to improve your bite, either for cosmetic or for a combination of cosmetic and medical reasons.

While it is no longer uncommon to see adults wearing braces or retainers, most doctors prefer teenage patients because their bodies change and heal faster. For the teeth to function their best, they must sit in the position they were designed to occupy. If your mouth is too small to accommodate all those teeth (This is not unusual), if your bite mismatches, if your teeth miss each other in their attempt to chew and grind food, you are probably a candidate for some type of orthondontia. Its aim is to make sure the jaws and teeth work together and that the pressure of chewing is evenly distributed throughout your mouth. Cosmetic matters come second.

Overcrowding is the biggest problem most orthodontists see: if the teeth aren't lined up correctly, there just isn't enough room in the mouth for those thirty-two pearly-whites. The teeth don't know the area is overpopulated, so they come up anyway, pushing and shoving relentlessly to get some sort of ground in your gums. Teeth get pushed sideways or aren't allowed to grow up and out properly (hence the Dracula effect), which also allows plaque to build up in the crevices between the teeth and gums.

To make room for the teeth, the orthodontist may extract a back tooth, or he may apply braces or a retainer. Braces are fixed in the mouth for a period of time and apply the most force, therefore effecting the most change. Retainers rely on the dedication of their owner to achieve change.

Braces work by exerting pressure on the teeth so that they are moved on their roots to a slightly different position in the mouth. The orthodontist may tighten the braces at each checkup, for progress in doing their job. When I was going to school, it was very "in" to wear braces, and I wanted them because my best friend had them, but my dentist wouldn't give them to me. Now I need braces, but I haven't decided if I can endure them at thirty-three years of age, even though many adults now find them acceptable.

It really is best just to get it over and done with. There will never be a "right" time for braces. But nowadays, you won't be the only one among your peers sporting them, no matter what your age.

In days gone by (only twenty years ago—could that be ancient history?) there was only one kind of braces. Not anymore!

Now there are plastic braces, less conspicuous than their metal counterparts, and what they call "invisible" braces. These aren't truly invisible, they are just placed *behind* the teeth instead of around them. Invisible braces take longer to work their magic, but are especially good for people who need only mild corrective power.

Another type of invisible correction is offered by the Crozat Technique, in which a removable wire is fitted around the molars and behind the front teeth. This widens the dental arch, making a little extra room for teeth that may otherwise have a tight squeeze. Sometimes the Crozat wires are used along with traditional braces. Either way, the wire method makes brushing your teeth more difficult and needs constant checking to make sure the wires are in the right place.

If the doctor decides the amount of rearranging your teeth need is not as drastic, he may recommend other techniques.

The retainer is a plastic device made for each individual, for either upper or lower (or both) teeth, that can be worn for differing time periods—depending on your needs. Retainers are used to stabilize tooth movement after braces come off. You remove the retainer for eating (which is why so many people lose their retainers) and proper cleaning. And for serious kissing. The effectiveness of a retainer depends on your personal discipline—if you cheat and don't use the device, you cheat yourself and your bite will never completely change.

Clean and care for your retainer per your orthodontist's instructions—don't play with your retainer, then put it back into your mouth.

There are several types of removable appliances like the "Hawley" or the "Crozat"; your doctor will recommend one according to your needs.

Headgear treats buck teeth in conjunction with braces and includes a strap that fits around the head and attaches to a mouthpiece. Depending on the severity of your problem, you may sleep with the headgear or wear it all the time. The more you wear it, the faster the results.

There are some important pointers to remember when deciding about orthodontic appliances. First of all, get a second opinion, just as you would for an important medical decision. Check the dentist's reputation. Do you know others who have used him? Were they satisfied? What kind of problems did they encounter, if any? Be sure to select someone who specializes in your particular problem; that way you know he has the requisite experience. Don't go to someone who promises to have you in and out in a jiffy. It takes time to move teeth correctly. Too much pressure too fast can loosen roots, which can lead to future trouble. It is important for your dentist or specialist to spend time with you, to understand and treat your problem. If the doctor says he'll have to extract some teeth, don't just acquiesce; get additional opinions. Always try to find a way to keep your teeth (even the wisdom teeth) if your mouth can accommodate them. Check out each doctor's reputation carefully. Use the best you can afford!

CAPS, BRIDGES, FALSIES

We've all heard about capped teeth because we know that many movie stars with perfect teeth (the kind we all wish we had been born with) really have caps. Capping involves filing down the real tooth and replacing it with a "cap," or "crown." Caps transform jagged, imperfect, broken or discolored teeth into the envy of all. Caps are costly, but there are several newly developed methods for rebuilding teeth that are less expensive and often don't necessitate filing the original away. No matter which route you take, be sure the color of the newly capped teeth matches the surrounding ones.

■ *Bonding:* Bonding is quick, painless and much less expensive than caps. The tooth is acid-etched to roughen up the surface texture (much like filing a nail before applying the fake) so that the new material will have nooks and crannies to adhere to. Then the tooth is rebuilt to the new shape with a resin and finished off with a glaze. The bonding material is translucent and comes in a variety of colors so the dentist can paint your new tooth to match your existing ones. There is little evidence bonding will hurt your teeth (the one being covered or the ones next to it), and it doesn't go into the gum, so there's no chance of infection. A broken tooth can be fixed via bonding, or a crooked one can be made to appear straight.

■ *Tooth painting:* A colored enamel can be painted onto teeth to brighten them up. This is strictly cosmetic. If you make public appearances or are on television, tooth painting may enhance your looks. Stained teeth also look better when painted.

■ *Bleaching:* Mostly replaced by bonding, bleaching is now done on teeth that darken after root-canal work. Vital (healthy) teeth are rarely bleached anymore.

■ *The Maryland Bridge:* When several teeth are missing ("All I want for Christmas is my two front teeth"), dentists traditionally create a bridge—a series of false teeth attached to a metal brace or plate which is then implanted in the mouth and attached to sound surrounding teeth, or which slides into and out of the mouth much like a retainer with teeth on it. The Maryland Bridge (invented at the University of Maryland) works by attaching metal wings to porcelain teeth to create a bridge which is then bonded to the adjacent teeth. There's no damage to the good teeth, and the procedure is painless.

■ *Implants:* Implants are used only in extreme cases, and the medical condition in the patient must be right. (Implants are not for patients who are heavy drinkers, who are diabetic or who have heart or kidney problems. Because only 50 percent of implants are successful, the patient must have good healing abilities.) The implant, a fake tooth, or series of teeth, is attached to an "anchor," which is surgically placed into the bone beneath the gums. The anchor is a post to which the new teeth (or single tooth) are fastened.

PREGNANCY AND TOOTH CARE

One of the first people to be able to tell if you are pregnant is your dentist. He or she may know even before you do! Often the gums change, and even little "P.T.s"—pregnancy tumors—will sprout. They are small swollen areas of gum that may bleed easily and should not be irritated by the tongue for curiosity's sake. P.T.s are not malignant and will go away a few weeks after your baby is born. Your dentist will prescribe a medicinal mouthwash or gargle to help keep the area free of infection.

Even if brushing your teeth makes you gag (not uncommon during pregnancy), continue to brush frequently. Gum massage should also be continued. Don't be alarmed at a reddening of the gums; it's only pregnancy gingivitis and will go away after the baby is born.

Prenatal tooth care begins with pregnancy—it's never too soon to start taking care of your child's teeth. A university study has shown that if the mother drinks fluoridated water, the fetus will develop stronger teeth. (If your community doesn't have fluoridated water, ask your doctor about vitamins with fluoride added—for you and your newborn child.) Once your baby is born, give him fluoride in vitamin drops. Even though babies have no teeth, and baby teeth come and go in a matter of a few years, your child's dental future is determined in the crucial period between conception and his sixth birthday.

LIP TIPS

To keep your lips in their best shape, take care of them all year around.

■ Don't lick or bite your lips, even if they feel dry or itchy.

■ Don't peel the dry skin on your lips.

■ Remember that change of climate is hard on lips. In winter, make sure they are covered with lip balm before you apply lipstick. Always apply lip balm at night. Balm should contain camphor and menthol in a petroleum base.

■ Use a lip gloss, balm or ointment even if you don't use lipstick, and use it all year round—especially outdoors in sun or cold.

■ Constantly reapply lipstick and balm, even though you may not feel your lips need it.

■ Never reapply new lipstick on top of old; it will look crusty and crackled. Clean your lips with makeup remover, or at least blot off old lipstick, first.

■ Lips are sensitive to hot and cold. Hot drinks can be drying, so beware of steaming coffee, tea and hot chocolate.

■ If out in sun or elements, layer lipstick treatments every hour (more frequently if necessary).

■ Pamper injured lips at night with a layer of balm or ointment.

■ Lip surgery can change the shape of your lips, but makeup tricks will suffice if you simply don't like your lip contour. I don't recommend surgery unless you have a serious lip problem. (Surgeons can make lips smaller, but not bigger.)

HERPES AND COLD SORES

Herpes has been the "hot" media disease these past few years, so almost everyone has some knowledge of the herpes simplex virus. There are two types—Viruses 1 and 2. Type 1 is usually confined to the facial area and is officially called "oral herpes." Type 2 occurs in the genital area. You can also get herpes in your eyes, which is extremely painful but, luckily, not too common. Experts estimate that 98 million people in the United States suffer at some time from herpes sores on or in their mouths. That's almost half the population!

Also called "cold sores" and "fever blisters," herpes lesions are harmless to the basically healthy person—they go away in a few days without causing scars. They can, however, spread to someone else (The germs are carried in saliva)—so refrain from kissing and other acts of intimacy while you have a sore. Generally there isn't enough pain to warrant medical treatment, but aspirin or Tylenol may be helpful. A saltwater mouthwash will help clean lesions inside the mouth.

If you have several lesions or frequent recurrences, see a doctor!

Having Type 1 herpes does not mean you will automatically get Type 2. To get the genital variety of herpes you must come in contact with someone who is carrying that type of the virus.

OTHER PROBLEMS

If you have sores, bumps or swelling in your mouth, see your dentist immediately. Only he or she can diagnose properly. Any condition that remains unchanged (or gets worse) over a forty-eight-hour period deserves attention.

MOUTH EXERCISES

Many exercise and fitness books have chapters, or entire texts, devoted to the exercise you should do to keep your face "in shape." These consist of saying the vowels of the alphabet, making faces like a clown or puckering up like Lolita and going kiss-kiss.

I find such antics ridiculous. And harmful to the face.

Stand in front of a mirror and do these exercises. See how many tiny lines form as you scrunch your face up. Doing face exercises actually creates lines!

So give yourself a break: exercise your body; care for your face.

Six

Eyes

THE EYES HAVE IT

The jukebox hisses as it drops the latest platter into place and spins a tale of a siren with "Bette Davis eyes." Every woman in the room is aware of the lyric. Those with Bette Davis eyes try to make their partners see the similarity. Those without them wonder whether they might instead have Elizabeth Taylor or Brooke Shields eyes. Few are content with their own.

No wonder. The eyes are the window of the soul! They are the focal point of the face. If the eyes have it, the world knows. If the eyes are dull and lifeless, or even if they're badly made up or lost in a sea of hair, the face loses impact. Eyes should be a person's best asset.

Your eyes are delicate, sensitive, perishable and not particularly replaceable. Not just the most expressive, they are one of the most important organs in the body.

EYEGIENE

I always call eye hygiene eyegiene because it makes consummate good sense, even if it looks silly written out. Because the eyes are one of the organs that must perform a vital function while simultaneously accommodating makeup and modern beautifying techniques, taking care of them is essential.

- Keep makeup away from the inside of your eyes at all times.
- Keep all makeup tools impeccably clean.
- Never borrow another person's eye makeup or eye-makeup tools. (Several class-

mates of mine did this once, and each went home with a severe case of pinkeye that ended up costing about $100 in medical bills and a week of school—right before finals, no less—just because they wanted to "try" a new shade of eyeliner that looked good on Tina before spending $4. Now, that's a case of false economy!)

■ Never use the eye makeup in displays in department and drug stores on your face—test on your hand to see shade or texture. You never know what germs the person before you had, and eye diseases like conjunctivitis (also called pinkeye) are highly contagious.

■ Close your eyes when you remove your eye makeup.

■ Use a cream or makeup remover to take off eye makeup. Then, to be sure you have gotten all excess oils, circle the eye area with a fresh piece of cotton moistened with water and gently wipe lashes. Do one eye at a time. The best creams are the ones sold as eye-makeup remover or cream for makeup removal. A liquid (like baby oil) will run into your eyes and burn, blur vision and invite infection.

■ Remove eye shadow and liner first, then mascara.

■ After removing all makeup, dip a cotton ball into cold water, squeeze out the excess and pat against the eye area to get off trace oils from the makeup remover. Check to make sure no specks or mascara flecks remain. Blot dry.

■ Do NOT sleep with your eye makeup on, even if you are involved in a hot love affair. (Okay, you're planning to ignore this piece of advice? At least do yourself this *one* favor: apply fresh, clean eye makeup before bed. This trick actually came from my eye doctor. He stresses that it's not a great idea, it's merely *better* than going to bed with old makeup on your eyes. It's still *best* to take it off.)

■ If makeup-removal creams irritate your skin, use a detergent-free cleansing bar instead. Moisten a piece of cotton, not a ball, run it across the cleansing bar, wipe and cleanse your eyes, then rinse with another water-soaked piece of cotton.

■ Avoid eye drops; don't get dependent on them for removing redness. If your eyes are red, they're red for a reason. Find out why and treat the problem, not the symptom. Monica used eye drops regularly, but her eyes seemed to get worse and worse. The worse they got, the more drops she used. Her eye doctor suggested she discontinue the drops. Two weeks later Monica's eyes were clear. She had had no need for the drops to begin with. The moral being: your eyes can become accustomed to using clarifying drops they don't need. So don't start using them!

■ Use only sable eye-makeup brushes. They are not as expensive as they sound, and they are the *softest*, so you won't get an irritation. Invest in a good set and care for them with regular cleanings in Barbicide, and they will last you many years and be well worth the price.

■ Don't wear contact lenses if your eyes feel tired or sensitive. Wear your regular glasses for a day or so, until they feel better. Have your lenses professionally cleaned and checked every six to eight months to make sure no damaging scratches exist.

TAKING CARE

If you study the human skeleton, you'll see that no bones touch the eyes or support the skin surrounding them. The eyes fit into sockets and do their work through a series of muscles and ligaments. Bones support your cheeks, your chin and your forehead, but there is nothing underneath to hold up the skin around your eyes. You must therefore be especially careful that this skin does not fall into those sockets to give you old, tired or droopy-looking eyes.

There are four main rules that will keep your eyes at their best if you observe them from your teen years on:

1. Use an eye cream every morning, not at night. It's during the day that your expression lines form, because that's when you use your eyes. Use twice a day if you reapply makeup. An eye cream is more concentrated than a moisturizer. Since the skin around your eyes has no oil glands, a light cream like a moisturizer is not sufficient there. A heavy-textured cream is required—and I recommend that you get used to it. Having what you like is not always the most beneficial. Eye cream really adheres to the under-eye area, helping to keep skin soft and supple so lines don't set in so readily. Try this test yourself, if you don't believe me: Scrunch up a piece of dry paper. Look at all the lines setting in. Now scrunch up a wet piece of paper. See the difference?

2. DON'T RUB makeup or cream into the eye area. It pulls the skin. Pat gently, from the outside of the eye inward. Be sure to start all the way to where crow's-feet occur: Look in the mirror and smile. Wherever you see little laugh lines around the eyes is where eye cream should be applied. Be sure not to go too close to lashes so no cream sticks to them and ends up in your eye.

3. Never sleep in your makeup. It can get into your eye and cause an infection. Break this rule as infrequently as possible.

4. *Be gentle* in applying makeup, removing it, giving yourself treatments around the eyes. Never get impatient, never panic. If you have a problem, panic can only make it worse.

If:

- you get cotton on your upper eyelashes—brush it off with a wet Q-Tip in an upward motion; brush downward for the bottom lashes.
- you get makeup in your eye—flush it out with eyewash (like Blinx or boric acid) or water. Don't try to stab with your finger.
- you stab your eye with a mascara wand—rinse the eye with eyewash or water, gently. Do not press or rub. Apply a cold-water compress or ice cubes for a few minutes. Keep the eye closed. If pain continues after ten minutes, call your ophthalmologist for an urgent appointment. (Tell the nurse what has happened to you.)
- you get an eyelash in your eye—gently fish it out with a wet Q-Tip.

GENETICALLY SPEAKING

A lot of the way your eyes look, see and age is a result of genetics—not cosmetics—and can be predicted by taking a look at your mother and other family members. The best bone structure for non-aging eyes is a prominent cheekbone, which is hereditary. Oily skin also ages less quickly than dry, and skin type is often hereditary. Bad vision also is commonly genetic. And squinting just makes lines worse! Many people need glasses but are too vain to wear them and force themselves to squint. It helps you see a little bit better, but forces you into a thousand enduring frown lines. If you need glasses, wear them, or investigate contact lenses, but *don't squint*! And be sure to wear sunglasses when you go out into the bright outdoor light.

There are some ways to fight heredity and aging with plastic surgery (see page 152), but it's preferable to avoid these tactics by taking care of your skin and eyes on a day-to-day basis.

GLASSES

There are two ways of looking at glasses:

A) as a disaster or

B) as a fashion accessory to your clothes and image. I think you'll find that once you choose Outlook B, you'll like your glasses and yourself in them.

I got my first pair of glasses early—in third grade. My father had bad eyesight, so it was really just a matter of time before his problem became mine, but in those days I was more concerned with peer pressure. Not being able to see clearly embarrassed me. My best friend had hawkeyes and there I was, called on to read from the blackboard, and all I could see was a blur. I would wander around not recognizing people I knew. Often others mistake "blind bats" for "big snobs." When you can't see clearly, you don't return those friendly smiles or winks.

Since then, I've spent a lot of time trying on frames and buying glasses. I've made a few mistakes (everyone does) over the years, but each time I've learned a little bit better what's right for my face, my fashion look and my lifestyle.

Buy as many pairs as you can afford. If you can afford two pairs, they should be a clear-lens pair and prescription sunglasses. If you can afford more, have one pair for every day and one pair for evening or dress-up occasions. Beyond that, you can begin to coordinate frames to the basic colors in your wardrobe. Over the last couple of years, I have collected some red frames, some pale pink pearly frames, a tortoiseshell pair and a metal pair.

When you go to pick out glasses, keep some of these facts in mind:

■ Go alone. If you bring people along, they will all have opinions. If you don't trust your own judgment, think about the frames overnight and go back to the shop later. Don't ever make a decision on frames based on someone else's taste.

■ Don't try to make a quick decision. You should feel comfortable enough to try on every pair of frames in the shop. Think about what the shape is doing to your face. Is it making your eyes look close-set? Do the frames extend well beyond your face? (They shouldn't.) Does the shape give you a lift, or do they curve down? Don't feel obliged to buy a pair just because you've spent an hour experimenting. That's part of the business. If you are pressured to buy, go to another shop!

■ Make sure your glasses are not too heavy. Nowadays, not only do they have plastic lenses, but you can get plastic frames as well. The glasses should sit lightly on your nose and ears and look weightless on your face. Frames that weigh too much leave dents on your nose and can break capillaries; headaches also come from weighty or pinching frames. When you try on frames, they have no lenses in them, so it's hard to estimate how heavy they will become. Remember that the larger the frame, the larger the lens and therefore the heavier the end result.

■ If you are choosing one all-purpose pair of glasses, choose a frame that is most likely to blend with all your clothes. Certain types of frames give certain looks. Clear Lucite, pink or metal may work best for you.

■ White frames usually look seasonal and casual. Unless you live in California, they are good only for summer wear.

■ Silver is harsh on fair skin; try white, off-white or bronze.

■ Pink may sound like a stupid color, but try it—it usually blends well and may be nearly invisible on your face.

■ Tortoise and brown shades are usually intellectual-looking. If this is too austere or preppy for you, warm up the effect with a tinted or colored lens.

■ Ask your opthalmologist about tints. Some people like tinted lenses for a fashion look, but tints can be harsh on your eyes for twenty-four-hour wearing. Get a firm medical opinion *before* you spend the money to have a tint put into your glasses. (A tint can always be bleached out, but you'll pay to have it put in.)

■ Also ask about a special coating that goes on plastic lenses to prevent scratching. Your optometrist can give you a special mailing envelope to send out your old glasses for this treatment. New glasses can be treated when they are made if you specify.

■ Have your eyes checked once a year for any changes.

SUNGLASSES

Everyone's eyes are naturally light-sensitive, so sunglasses are a help to all—even to those who do not wear prescription lenses. While you will not damage your eyes by going out in bright light, you will put strain or stress on them and force yourself to squint

—which is a no-no. You can find sunglasses in a wide variety of colors, styles and prices. To sort it all out, try to remember:

■ Pick sunglasses as you would a cosmetic. Go for the middle price range, weeding out the most and least expensive.

■ Browns, grays and greens for lens colors offer the most protection. Blue is pretty but not as effective; pinks and reds are distorting.

■ Never buy glasses with a lens darker than you need. You will get "hooked" on the density and keep needing darker and darker lenses. Different people need different shading, depending on their eye sensitivity.

■ Hold up the sunglasses to light and make sure the two sides match.

■ You should not be able to see your eyes clearly when you look at yourself in the mirror.

■ Sunglasses should fit your lifestyle. If you spend a lot of time at the beach and aren't careful, maybe you'll need several pairs of inexpensive glasses. If you are careful with your glasses or need a prescription pair, designer sunglasses may be what you have in mind.

■ Choose sunglasses to suit your face shape the same way you would regular eyeglasses.

■ While light-sensitive glasses are available, I don't think they work very well. Some find it convenient to have one pair of glasses that automatically darken when you go into bright light, but they don't get either dark enough in the sun or light enough in darker rooms, so I don't think they are worth the extra money.

CONTACT LENSES

So advanced is the state of the contact-lens art that it's rare to find a person who cannot wear one type or another. I got my first pair when I was in high school. Another girl in the class had preceded me in this adventure, covering her beautiful blue eyes with a pair of green lenses. At first I thought her eyes were startlingly beautiful and wanted contacts just like hers. Then one day I saw her outside and the angle of light hit those phony green lenses, turning her eyes into traffic lights.

When I did get my lenses, I got a clear lens with just enough tint so I could find it if I dropped one. Which didn't happen often because I seldom wore them; they were just too uncomfortable to bear. My first experience with contacts was unfortunate. I returned to being a blind bat, wearing my glasses only in emergencies.

It took me another four years to get up the courage to try again. My second attempt, when I was in college, was bliss from the beginning. I've hardly had any trouble since. But I did have one ironic realization. Before I got my lenses, I used to think that all the people who walked on Fifth Avenue in New York (where I grew up) were beautiful. Then I got my contact lenses and for the first time saw how they really looked—like ordinary people. What a blow to my fantasy!

Once I got my contact lenses, my whole

self-image began to change. Being able to see (at last) was wonderful, and not wearing glasses gave me an exhilarating confidence.

If you think you are a candidate for contact lenses, talk to your eye doctor about the many options. Here is a chart of some of the possibilities.

Contact Lenses

Hard lens	A rigid piece of plastic with an inflexible curve which is fitted to match the curve of your cornea. Can be cleaned in a few seconds, need to be polished once or twice a year. Lenses will cost $200–250; medical care is additional.
Gas-permeable	Not soft lenses, but not as hard as "hard" lenses, gas-permeable lenses allow for oxygen to get in and out, which makes them more comfortable to many. Cost is $250–$350, plus medical care.
Soft lens	Made of pliable, waterlike plastic, soft lenses allow oxygen in and out. However, because they are almost all water, they demand sterilization and special handling. They are not for careless or lazy people. Lenses $70–$150; medical care extra.
Extended-wear	Known as the twenty-four-hour lenses, extended-wear are soft lenses that are meant to *stay* in the eye for up to two weeks. Lenses are expensive ($300) and need constant medical attention. Look for a doctor whose fee includes *all* the help you may need.

Contact-Lens Beauty Tips

■ Don't wet your hard lenses with saliva. That's downright unsanitary.

■ Keep your hands clean when dealing with eyes and lenses.

■ If a hard lens pops out, try to scoop it up with a sheet of paper rather than your fingers.

■ Don't be too lazy to clean your lenses properly.

■ Don't wear your lenses for too many hours, if your eyes are red or irritated, if you don't get enough sleep or have been up all night.

■ Put lenses in before you put on makeup. (Insert lenses, wait a few minutes for them to settle, then apply makeup.)

■ Don't sleep in your lenses unless they are the kind made for twenty-four-hour wear.

■ If you go to a salon for a facial, bring a case for storing your lenses.

■ If you travel on a plane, carry a small bottle of wetting solution in your handbag. The higher altitude causes the fluid in your eyes to dry, and you'll be very uncomfortable. Try using artificial tears (Many brands are available).

EYE DISTRACTIONS

No one's eyes look their best all the time. Your eyes are hypersensitive—to the amount of sleep you've had, to air pollution, to makeup and a hundred other factors, many of which you cannot even see. If you're prone to puffiness, circles, redness or constant infections, try some of these tips:

1. Make sure all makeup is removed properly before you sleep.
2. Use fragrance-free cosmetics and eye-makeup products.
3. Sleeping with night cream on the skin around your eyes may cause puffiness if it creeps into the eyes.
4. Cold compresses will reduce puffiness. Allow time in your schedule in the morning and before special evening dates to apply a compress. Try resting on a slant board with your head higher than your feet for five or ten minutes.
5. If you have a water-retention problem, stay away from salty foods.
6. Too much alcohol can cause puffiness and circles.

ALLERGIES

You can become allergic to anything, so suddenly that a product you have used and adored may, in effect, turn on you and have to be discontinued. Your skin may be sensitive; you may have had an allergy since childhood or you may develop a brand-new one overnight. All things are possible and need the proper treatment.

- If you have a history of allergies, use allergen-tested makeup and fragrance-free products.
- Use fresh products; throw out the old and the used. Change mascara every three months whether it's all been used or not.
- Avoid eye products that have sparkles in them—these are usually made from mica or fish scales. Sensitive eyes are more prone to an allergic reaction; choose matte colors.
- Use matte cream shadow or pencil rather than powders because they won't flake off into the eyes.
- If you have itchiness, don't scratch. Discontinue makeup immediately. If the problem continues more than forty-eight hours, call your eye doctor.
- Your problems may be seasonal or have to do with the air quality. If you are prone to allergies and have your choice of cities for college or jobs, investigate the weather conditions and air quality first.

OTHER EYE PROBLEMS

If you have red, itchy eyes, mucus in your eyes when you wake in the morning or just terribly tired eyes, you may have conjunctivitis. Highly contagious, this minor disease will not get better on its own. See your ophthalmologist for a prescription for drops or ointment, and follow the frequent-application schedule to rid yourself of the infection. If you apply the medicine only occasionally, it will take longer for your eyes to get better and you may need a stronger medication—and more trips to the eye doctor. (More $.)

Eye injuries should be treated immediately. Maribeth had her own elaborate way of applying mascara. She put it on in layers, let it dry, separated the lashes with a straight pin, then reapplied and repeated three or four times. One day the inevitable happened: the pin slipped and went right into her eye. After the immediate pain, Maribeth thought she was okay. It took about six hours for the pain to return and for her to realize she needed medical help. (See page 98.)

If you see flashing lightning or black dots, notify your eye doctor as soon as possible. This may indicate a problem.

EYE NEWS

Doctors are constantly using new technology to improve eyesight and correct eye problems. For people who are unable to wear glasses or contact lenses, there are two new types of surgery that are still in the experimental stages. Radial keratotomy is for extremely nearsighted people. The elongated eye is shortened surgically, restoring perfect vision. When performed on patients under age twenty-one, it requires parental permission, and *you should obtain several medical opinions* before venturing forth. An even newer technique allows surgeons to create a pocket in the cornea and insert a soft contact lens to correct vision. This too is experimental.

EYE TRICKS

Do your best always to make your eyes look their best and to show them off.

■ Keep your hair out of your eyes. Bangs may softly frame them, but don't hide behind hair.

■ If you wear glasses and want to make sure your conversation partner sees the real you, casually remove your glasses while you are talking and let him (or her) have the full effect *sans* plastic.

■ Be photographed without your glasses on, because the lens will cause light distortions or shadows. If you are appearing on TV, ask the cameraman if you are reflecting light. You may want to go it blind—especially if you are on a talk show and don't need to see anything. You can always place your glasses on top of your head. I know a CBS correspondent who wears contact lenses to correct his myopia and then wears tortoise frames without lenses in them to keep his scholarly image.

■ If allergies prevent you from wearing eye makeup, investigate eyelash dyes to see if you can tolerate them. If not, keep all your other makeup soft; bright face colors will only make your eyes look plainer. I have a client who cannot bear any eye makeup (including dye) because of sensitive skin. She has great posture, always coordinates her clothes perfectly, has her hair arranged just so and uses eyeglass frames as fashion accessories. This woman is so put-together that you stare at her in appreciation of her visual splendor, never noticing that she has on only makeup base and a little blush-on.

■ Use sunglasses with various degrees of tint in them to cover up eyes that are bloodshot or under the weather. Never wear dark sunglasses indoors, though. Light fashion tints are available for school and work lighting. Discuss the light conditions with your ophthalmologist when you choose tints.

■ Get the sleep you need.

■ Protect your eyes whenever possible.

EYEBROWS

Eyebrows are a great indicator of character on a face and should not necessarily be made to conform to current trends. While there are certain styles that come into fashion—like the thin, fiercely plucked eyebrows of the 1930s, the thick, pointed eyebrows of the '50s and the unkempt brows of the '60s—most women like their eyebrows artfully to set off their eyes. Eyebrows are like a frame to the eyes and should be one continuous stroke, like an arch, not a distracting up-and-over angle. They should never close down an eye.

■ If your eyebrows have a natural shape (many people's do), go with the flow.

■ If you believe in the character of your eyebrows, stand by it. Don't pluck just to be like everyone else.

■ Don't tweeze above your brows—only underneath to shape them. Stray hairs are messy and should be plucked in order for your makeup to look right.

■ If your eyebrows need help and you don't know what to do, go to a salon for professional guidance. A professional pluck plus advice and lessons will only cost about $7.50.

■ Choose eyeglass frames that cover your eyebrows—you do not want two sets of lines showing above your eyes.

■ If your brows won't stay in line, even after they've been shaped, use a mustache wax or an eyebrow-wax wand to comb and style brows.

■ Brows should usually be a little lighter than your hair color. This opens up the eye area and draws attention to them. (Eyelashes should be darker.)

■ If there is a gap in the eyebrows, a pencil should be used to draw in the illusion of hair. Similarly, if the brow needs to be shaped, a pencil should be used to draw a natural looking brow shape onto the skin.

■ If the eyebrow's natural shape and fullness is correct, an old, dry mascara is the most effective means to color the brow. The mascara attaches to the brow hair, giving the brow a very natural look.

■ Do not shave your eyebrows.

■ Don't go overboard when you tweeze. Your eyebrow should begin over the corner of your eye; end at the end of your eye.

■ Disinfect tweezers with alcohol before

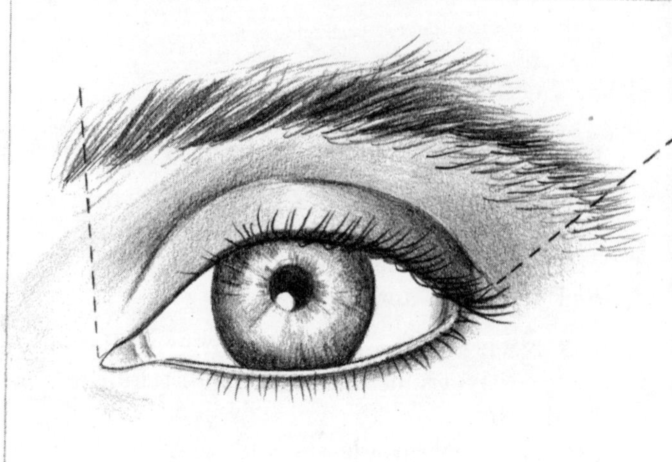

Shapeless brow: bushy, overpowering

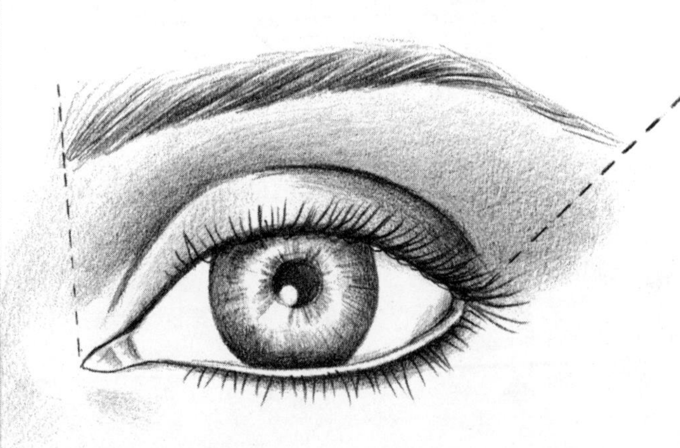

Proper brow shape: neat, gently arched

tweezing. Also dab a little alcohol on the brows with a cotton pad first. (Squeeze out excess so it doesn't drip into your eye!) After the tweezing, wash off the alcohol. Wait one half-hour before applying makeup so pores close up and no infection occurs.

EYELASHES

Eyelashes protect the eyes from incoming bits of dirt and debris and frame them dramatically. If you doubt the importance of eyelashes, leave one eye un–made-up, then apply mascara to the other. The difference is enormous! Even if you have thin pale eyelashes (like me), you can fool Mother Nature and your friends by using a dark mascara. While there are several colors on the market (Even a red one has been introduced), I think mascara should come just like the first Ford—in black only. The other colors are mere fashion gimmickry and don't perform as well as black does. No matter what your coloring, you can wear black mascara.

If you prefer, you can have your eyelashes dyed at a beauty salon. (*Never* attempt this at home.) Always have a tint test done ahead of time to make sure you are not allergic—test at least twenty-four hours before the dying date so you can be sure there will be no danger to your eyes. Dying is particularly nice for people with pale eyelashes whose lifestyle is so busy they cannot always be around makeup or mascara. I also recommend that men with pale eyelashes have theirs dyed.

If you're considering false eyelashes, I'd think twice. If you decide to try them, be *extremely* careful in applying the glue. Eyelids quickly build up a sensitivity to glue, and a drop in the eye can cause blindness! False eyelashes rarely look good up close, and the glue can weaken your own lashes. Unless you are appearing on stage, I think you can find a way to enhance your eyes without going through the time, expense and risk of fakes.

WORK OUT YOUR EYES

Eyestrain can bring on headaches and fatigue, so when you feel those well-known signs of burning, tearing or weariness, give your eyes a workout. Especially if you are keeping long hours (studying or working), you'll want to take breaks to relax your eyes as well as your shoulder and neck muscles.

Blinkout: Gently blink your eyes fre-

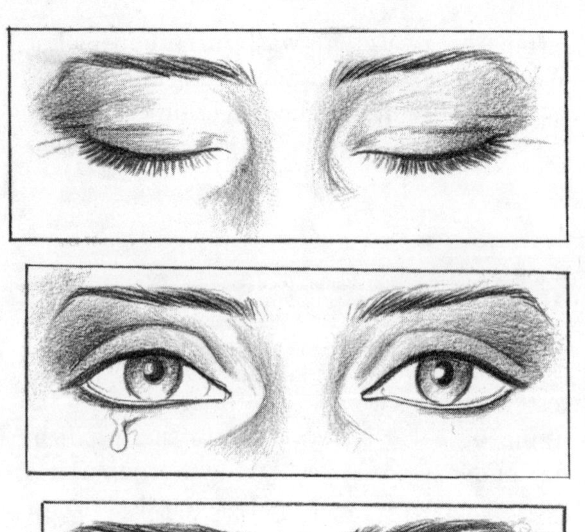

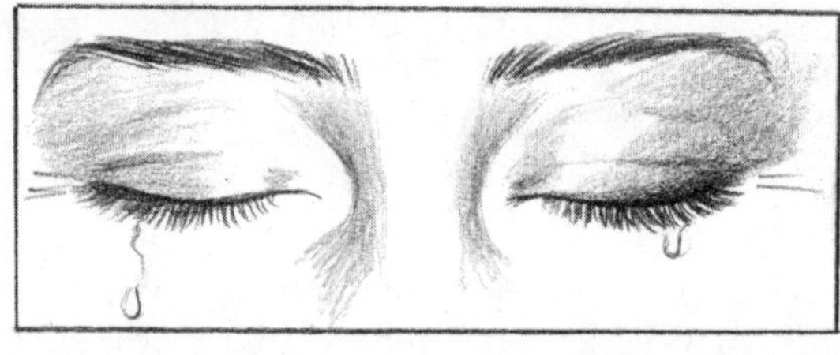

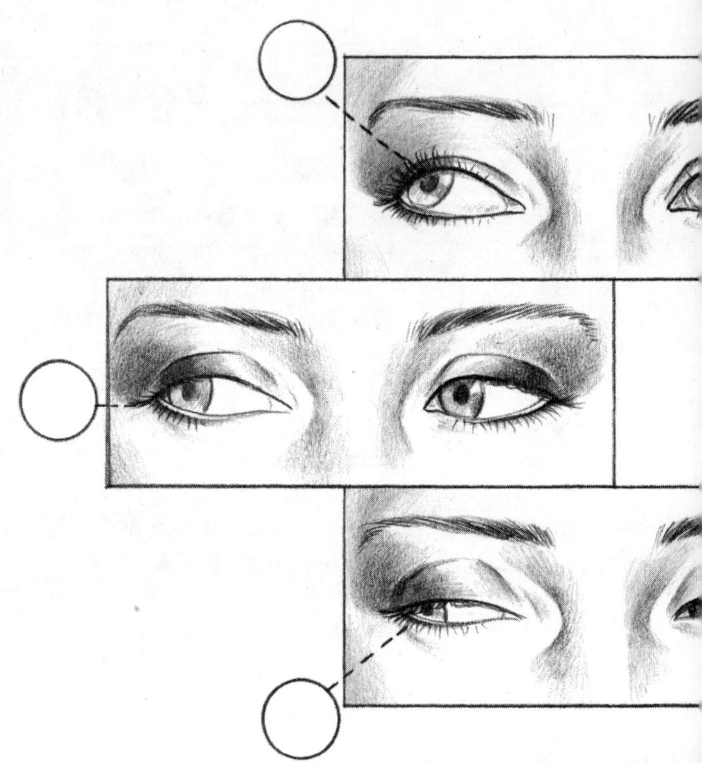

quently to gather up some tears beneath them. This lubricates eyes and gives them a rest. Stop the blinkout for a few seconds, then continue. Do five blinkouts.

Rollout: Slowly roll your eyes in circles. First right, then left.

Left-right: Hold index finger about six inches away from your eyes to the right. Both eyes should follow your finger as it moves from right to left and back again. Now repeat, moving your finger up and down.

Another easy eye saver that's especially helpful during long periods of close reading is *Lookout:* Take your eyes off your work and look out to a far point—out a window if possible. Look back and forth, about ten times or whenever your eyes need a break.

Remember, your eyes are precious. Give them the respect they deserve. If you have any problems, call your eye doctor. This is not a question for a cosmetologist.

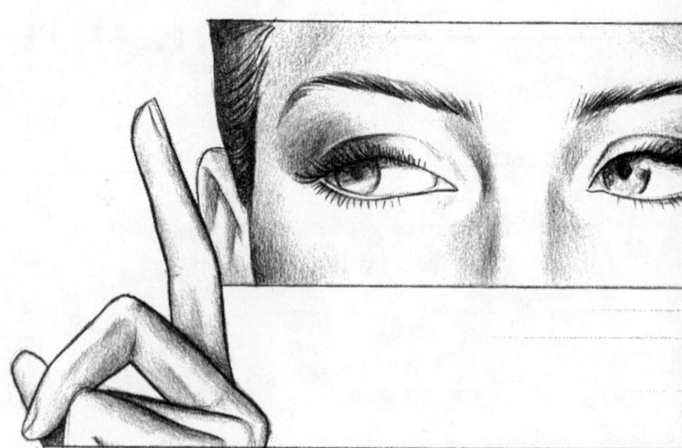

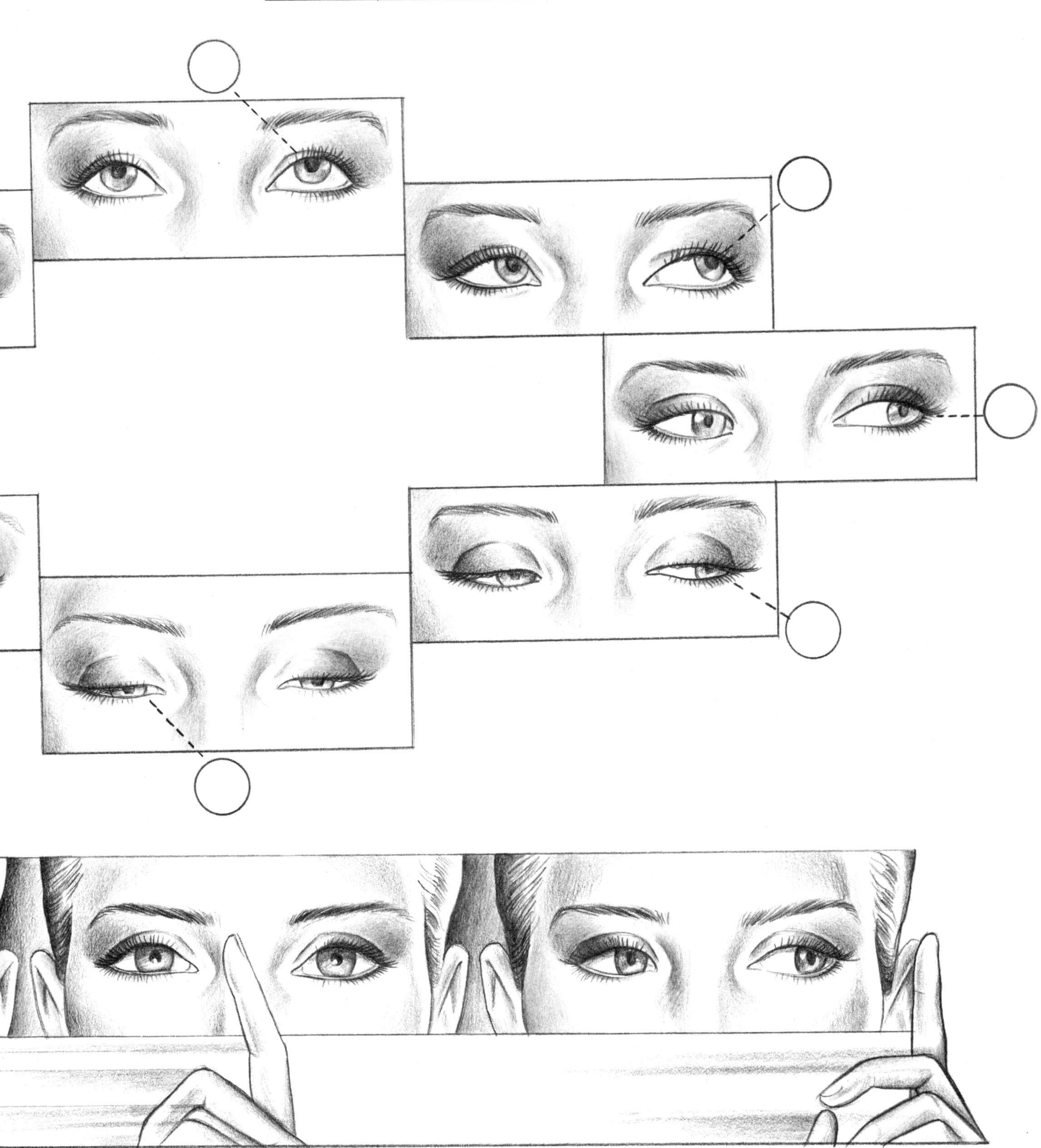

Seven

Hands and Feet

STICK 'EM UP

All right, this is a stickup. I want to see those hands and nails right now. That's what I thought.

Uneven nails.
Rough skin.
Chipped polish.
Pulled cuticles.
A hangnail.

And I thought you were a lady.

You don't have to be rich to have ladylike hands. You don't have to have polish on your nails or have a manicure—be it a salon or a home manicure. You just have to care. And caring takes time and effort. Considering the importance of your nails, the investment is well worthwhile—both cosmetically and psychologically.

Marina was twenty-four when she thought she'd met Mr. Right. "He was very rich," she told me, "and I wanted to fit in with his friends and his family and look like a lady. My idea of a real lady was a woman with long red nails that sparkled in the sunlight and clacked on the counter in stores when the salesgirl was too slow." With the help of a manicurist, Marina grew her nails out to the desired length and began coming in for a manicure every other week—all she could afford. After six months, she discovered that Mr. Right had a series of hang-ups and was more like Mr. Wrong, so her affair ended. But along the way, something else happened. "There was a big psychological boost. With the long red nails, I became the woman of my fantasies. I felt more sophisticated, more powerful, more grown-up. I actually felt like a woman instead of a girl. I stood up a little straighter, worked a little harder and felt a lot better about myself. The fifteen dollars a month I was spending on manicures brought me back more than fifteen dollars' worth of energy and confidence—and probably cash, because I worked harder and did get a raise. With those gorgeous nails I felt like *executive* material, and I proved it to my boss, too."

Hands are a dead giveaway of your self-esteem, your age and your profession. So give them the respect they deserve and let them work to your best advantage. Be sure to lavish sunblock on your hands when you go outdoors, especially for sports or a lot of sun—this will help prevent brown spots and "old" hands. There is no "face lift" for the hands, so take care of them now.

DETAILS COUNT

If you're the kind of person who knows the importance of details, then you're already aware of the impact your hands and feet make on your personal appearance. It's the little things that count, and when you meet someone for the first time—someone who is forced to judge you initially on appearances—you'll notice that sooner or later, eyes will fall to your hands. Remember poor Scarlett O'Hara, who was doing so well with Rhett in the Atlanta jailhouse until he took her hands in his, discovered them to be raw and blistered and realized she had been doing field work?

Just like Scarlett's, your hands—and your feet too (especially in summer)—say a great deal about you.

■ If your nails are long and perfectly manicured, your hands may give the impression you don't type, never touch dishes and, in fact, scorn hard work. While these hands are nothing to be embarrassed about, they give the wrong impression to an employer. (On a job interview, be sure to mention how sturdy your nails are, or make a joke about your fingers' being so fast on the computer or calculator that you never break a nail.)

■ If your nails are short and bitten off, never call attention to them with bright polish or dramatic flourishes. Keep your hands in low profile until you can get them into shape. A mere two weeks' time will rescue you from this embàrrassing situation.

■ If you play the guitar or do a job that requires constant use of your hands, let your fingernail length show that you work. Keep your nails manicured, but trimmed short. Clear or pale polish and a neat appearance say it all.

■ Don't apply false nails for a job interview, for a date, or to impress someone. Too many things can go wrong, and your movements will probably look unnatural. (You can actually feel the weight of false nails, and it is distracting.)

■ Don't play with your nails, pick or bite them or peel off the polish in public. Nervous? We all have our fidgety habits, especially under stress. Don't let the movement of your hands betray the butterflies in your stomach.

■ Don't clutter your fingers with rings or other distractions, especially if you are trying to convey the impression you are a working woman. If you are a debutante, heiress or princess or are auditioning for a similar role—be my guest.

■ If the nail polish on one finger chips, don't put a Band-Aid on it before a date or interview. Keep a bottle of nail polish in your handbag or car so you can touch up immediately. Or remove all the polish before the occasion. It's better to appear with no nail polish than with varnish chipped or half-peeled.

NAILS AND NUTRITION

What you eat is important in terms of how your nails look and last. Eating sensibly makes nails stronger and prevents them from becoming brittle or layering. You need sufficient amounts of food from the four food groups, as well as a small amount of vegetable oil each day. (You probably get this in salad dressing.) If you go on a crash or fad diet, you can bet you'll see a change in your nails. Despite the claims, gelatin does not seem to influence either the growth or the stability of nails. It isn't bad for them—it just doesn't seem to do much good. If you have white spots in your nails, it could indicate a calcium deficiency. Try a strong multi-vitamin; if that doesn't help, get some nutritional advice from an expert. Don't overdose on calcium and play home doctor.

NAIL FACTS

Nails are, of course, part of your body. They are made of layers of keratin, the same material that forms the hair shaft, and they grow out from what's called the matrix, which begins about where the first finger joint ends. (Which is why you always treat your nail up to the first joint.)

■ Nails must be kept clean, so wash them with a nail brush when you shower or bathe. If a nail brush doesn't remove dirt and grime, an orange stick will.

■ Dry nails are often the result of weather or water conditions. If you swim, do dishes or have unprotected hands out in the elements, moisturize them with lotion. Wear rubber gloves whenever possible, and avoid contact with harsh soaps, detergents and chemicals.

■ Polish remover is a chemical. Try not to use it more than once a week. Be sure to wash it off after use and let your nails breathe at least overnight before applying new polish.

■ Groom your nails in one way or another —be it an official "manicure" or your own ministrations—once a week. A complete home manicure is suggested, if you have time. If not, give yourself careful after-shower care by pushing back cuticles, using moisturizers and keeping nails carefully filed.

■ Buffing your nails increases circulation and makes them stronger. Buff once a week.

■ Exercise your hands. This keeps them strong and flexible and helps keep them expressive. (Hand models even take dance lessons focusing on their hands!) Keep a hand grip in the car to use while you are at stoplights—you can buy one at a sporting-goods store—or use an old tennis ball to strengthen your grip by alternately squeezing and releasing.

■ Protect your hands and nails with gloves.

■ Use the tips of your fingers rather than your nails whenever possible.

■ Nails grow an average of ⅛ inch per month. Nails on the same hand do not grow at an equal rate—the center nail grows faster.

■ Nails grow faster in summer and slow down in winter.

■ Nail growth and patterns may change during pregnancy . . . also after menopause.

■ The strength and shape of your nails is often hereditary.

■ Your nails probably have a natural length limit built into them, although sometimes you can extend that quotient. But don't be greedy. After a certain length, long nails only cause complications.

NAIL FLAIR

Almost everyone would choose to have long, strong nails if she could, but often this is not possible. No matter how stubborn your genes, though, you can still have attractive nails.

When you choose the nail look you want, it doesn't do much good to mimic a movie star or a high-fashion model. The nails that will look best on your hands are ones that fit your personality, your job and your lifestyle.

Nail shapes are largely a matter of fashion. Square nails were a big look in the 1970s when everyone wanted to look like Cher. Now more naturally shaped, slightly rounded nails are popular. Pointy nails haven't been in for decades, and nails of varying lengths went out with the French Revolution. (So much for King Louis' idea of having an exaggerated pinkie nail for scratching at the door instead of knocking.) I personally think that ovals will always be right, regardless of fashion.

You should see a change in your nails every week, which is rewarding if you are watching them grow out. If you are just starting this process, keep your nails clean and healthy with weekly manicures, care for them properly but try not to be obsessed with them. Staring at them will not make them grow any faster. Protein-based polishes and nail hardeners will help fragile nails. Hand lotion (or even eye cream, with its extra-duty enrichers) will help nails, as will special nail nutrients. Be sure to keep cuticles soft. Apply cream nightly, and massage it in gently. (There are several brands on the market.) Wrap manicures or Juliette-style conditioners with fibers in them can strengthen weak nails until they grow in stronger. Glue on your nails is unhealthful and will not make them stronger in the long run.

Choose your nail shape *after* the nails have grown in. Just let them rise from your fingertips slowly and gracefully. Many times the nails simply stop growing at a certain length. This could be your signal to leave well enough alone and maintain this length, or you may want to get professional help to push your nails to new heights. Shannon had nails that grew to a nice length. They were healthy and always well cared for. But to Shannon the grass was greener on her friends' hands and she craved long nails. With weekly manicures and the use of rubber gloves for household tasks, Shannon was able to add a quarter-inch to her regular length and get a bonus as well: her new length proved to be stronger than ever.

THE MANICURE

The main difference between a professional and an at-home manicure is not a matter of putting on the polish, but a matter of the care your hands actually get. Putting on polish neatly is a skill you can probably learn well enough to get through life without ever having another person do it for you. But taking the time to really *care* for your nails the way a pro does is something else again.

The Home Manicure

If you have a regular beauty night, then a home manicure fits right into your schedule. If you don't, you'll probably be happier setting aside a specific time for it. Many working women find they can give themselves a better manicure at the office than at home, so if you have the time and the supplies, and your boss doesn't mind (or notice), that's one alternative. If you work all day and come home to a house filled with children, you may indeed find office hours the only chance you get for your nails to dry properly. (If you go to sleep with "tacky"—somewhat damp—nails, you'll wake with sheet presses on them.)

Whether it's at home or at work, try for a regular schedule, and give yourself an hour at the least, an hour and a half if you can. While the manicure doesn't take very long, you *do* need a lot of drying time.

Assemble all your supplies in one place, be it bathroom, desk or bureau. You should have ready before you begin:

- small cereal bowl
- base coat, topcoat and polish
- polish remover and cotton balls
- cuticle remover
- orange stick
- nail clipper
- emery board (not metal nail file)
- hand lotion or cream

Steps:

1. Fill the bowl with warm, sudsy water and soak one hand at a time. Towel-dry the hand, then push back cuticle with towel; do not cut it.

2. If any of your nails have grown *too* long, clip them to an even length.

3. Now shape nails with the emery board. Move it only toward the center of the nail, using the fine side of the board. Shape nails to be softly rounded or oval.

4. Apply cuticle softener, leave on for five–ten minutes (no longer—it's a chemical, remember) and push back the cuticles again with orange stick.

5. With cuticles done, apply hand cream from nail tips to elbows. Massage in circular motion as you go. Particularly work on the area from fingertip to first joint of each finger, as this is where the nail grows from.

6. If you are mending or patching, do so now. If I have a serious break, I forget about patching (It's always lumpy) and clip down all the other nails to the same length and start fresh. That way all your nails will grow back at approximately the same rate and they'll be good and strong.

7. If you are buffing, do so now (but not on patched nails). People with thin nails may not want to buff.

8. Apply base coat, then polish. Most of the time, two coats of polish are sufficient. If you are using the kind of base coat with fibers in it, you may want to apply a regular base coat over it to ensure smooth going when you put on the polish.

9. Let the polish dry to at least tacky—about fifteen minutes. Then, using an orange stick swathed in cotton, dip the stick into polish remover and clean up any spots on your fingers. Be sure you don't dent your polish or drip remover on your nails.

10. Apply topcoat or clear nail hardener and allow nails to dry and set.

The Salon Manicure

When you go to a salon for a manicure, the manicurist will follow many of the steps just outlined. Your part in the drama includes the following:

1. If you have any instructions for the manicurist, give them to her before she starts working on your hands. Tell her what you like, don't like and want for your nails. Say you're trying to grow them out, you like them squared off, you think they're too long or whatever else is on your mind. Finding a good manicurist is a lot like finding the right hairstylist.

2. It's not unusual for the client to provide her own nail polish. This way she has a bottle of it so she can touch up her nails herself. You can also buy a bottle of the color the manicurist gives you, if you use that shade often enough to warrant the expense.

3. If you want a nail hardener used as a topcoat, say so. If you want more than two coats of polish, say so.

4. Be prepared to pay for extra services. It is unlikely the manicurist will charge you extra for a third coat of polish, but she may charge if you request "moons" or special polishing techniques. Wrapping, repairs, porcelain nails and other fancy procedures always cost more.

5. Tip the manicurist 15 percent of her bill. If you have a standing or regular appointment, a Christmas gift or extra tip is *de rigueur*.

6. Be on time. Call if you are going to cancel—don't be a "no-show."

ADDED ATTRACTIONS

If your nails aren't all they should be, or could be, perhaps you're considering adding onto them. There are several methods, all with drawbacks. Your nail beds are alive, so anytime you cover them and don't allow them to breathe, you are asking them to suffocate a little.

Patti nails: invented by a dentist and named after his wife, Patti nails are false nails built over your own out of a mixture similar to what dentists use for fillings.

Wrapped nails: a technique by which tissue paper, silk or fabric is glued to and wrapped around the nails to strengthen them. Usually looks lumpy, and if glue is being applied to your nails—watch out, baby. Glue on your nails can seep through the nails and into the nail bed.

Porcelain nails: a type of Patti nail that is thinner and smoother.

I'm not a fan of any of these techniques, because they are basically bad for overall nail health, but the choice is yours.

NAIL TIPS

If you bite your nails, you should be able to stop within a week. It takes willpower and sometimes the use of a bad-tasting paint-on product that will burn your lips.

■ Your nails should be pink and healthy-looking. If they aren't, you could be showing the effects of smoking, drinking, bad health, too much polish or an allergy to any of the nail products you are using.

■ Weak nails will grow stronger if you clip them back regularly.

■ Your nails should go without polish for at least twenty-four hours. Let your nails breathe!

■ Wear rubber or plastic gloves for washing dishes, pots and pans, gardening, bleaching clothes and applying hair color.

■ If you have short or fat fingers (Yes, some people have pudgy fingers), apply nail polish down the center only, leaving a discreet margin between the cuticle and the polish. This little optical illusion will make your nails and fingers look a tad longer.

■ If you have ordinary hands, wear an ordinary color—go neither for flashy nor for mousy.

■ Pick polish that is flattering to your skin; do not match it to your clothes or your eyeglass frames. If your hands are too red, avoid red and pink tones—pick coral or orange or peach tones.

■ If you are getting married or participating in an event that will be photographed, do not wear a trendy polish. Years from now you will be embarrassed when friends start hooting, "What *color* is that on your nails?"

■ Nails have cycles too. They will invariably have long and short periods that are beyond your control.

■ Learn to use your hands properly to protect your nails.

HAND HOW-TOS

1. Learn to use the pads of your fingers rather than the tips.
2. If you have dial phones, exchange them for push-button, or use the eraser of a pencil to dial.
3. Reach out with your hands slightly flexed so your nails aren't in extreme jeopardy.
4. Your nails are not tools. Remove stains with a sponge; pry open lids with a can opener.

HAND CARE

Just as the TV commercials say, hands are a clear indicator of age. So if you're planning on fooling the public by taking good care of your face, you owe it to yourself to pamper your hands too.

Because the hands go through so many shocks—from weather to chemical variations—in one day, they toughen up rapidly. A person's occupation has a good bit to do with what his or her hands look like. People who play the guitar develop useful calluses on their fingertips; scientists in laboratories often develop tough skin that enables them to handle chemicals or temperatures normal hands would flinch at. But for most people, hand care is merely a matter of time, concern and the cost of a good hand lotion.

Consider your hands to begin at the elbow and end at your fingertips. Lather them with hand lotion every time you bathe and before bed. If your hands are in and out of water frequently, apply lotion more often.

Tiffany tells me the secret of her beautiful hands and long nails is the fact that she always carries a plastic bottle of hand lotion in her handbag and thinks nothing of massaging her hands five to ten times a day. She says her hands are not an obsession, but whenever she thinks about it, she just puts on more lotion.

Weather particularly affects the skin on the elbows and arms, so keep your body smooth and soft by extending your hand care elbow-ward. Scaly elbows may not be the end of the world, but when summer comes along and you go bare-armed, you'll know you look your best when your body is smooth.

Remember, hands give away age! Apply

hand cream nightly and daily to protect and maintain soft, youthful-looking skin. Use gloves while doing dishes; even though you would rather not be bothered, they do help. Keep your cuticles soft by applying cream and massaging nightly.

If you have old facial-care products that you aren't using or that may have been too oily for your face, you can use them up on your hands, knees and feet so they aren't wasted.

FROM TOE TO KNEE

Just as you consider your elbow part of your hand, be good to your feet and begin to think of your knee as a mere extension of your toes. Since you probably shave your legs, your calves are in need of tender loving care. And knees always need all the help they can get—like elbows, they have a tendency to be less than charming when neglected.

One of the questions a lot of people ask me is why they should spend the time and money to take care of their feet when so few actually see them. There are several reasons:

1. *Your health.* Your feet support your whole body. They are the basis of your career as an active person; if you have problems with them you will tire easily, suffer pain and definitely be a grump. You can also throw your posture out of whack and ruin your back.

2. *Your looks.* During the winter you may be the only person who sees your feet. During the summer, they are constantly on display in sandals, open-toed shoes; in sports and beach activities. If you ignore your feet for six months while they nestle in your red rubber rain boots with the fake sheepskin lining, they will not look their best come the first day you fall prey to spring fever and long to run your toes through the clover in the park. Year-round foot care is to your best advantage.

3. Even if you *are* the only person who sees your feet, *you* count! It will make you feel a lot better to have well-groomed feet. This is where psychological aspects of beauty come in. Listen to what Melissa told me: "I was feeling really sorry for myself because I didn't have a boyfriend and all my friends were going home for the holidays or doing something special with their boyfriends and I was just a lump with no place to go. So I treated myself to one of those half-day beauty plans, and believe it or not, the part that had the best effect on me was the pedicure. I thought a pedicure was silly—I mean, I didn't even have a boyfriend to *see* my toes, so I had no one to impress—but it was part of the price for the day, and they don't give you your money back if you skip phases of the plan, so they gave me this big fancy pedicure. Not only did it feel fantastic, but for about a month afterward, every time I looked down and saw my beautiful toes and their sparkling color winking up at me, it made me smile. I felt glamorous, and sexy, and rich and special. Just because a tiny part of me was bright red. Now I'm a believer!"

4. A home pedicure is a great way to pamper yourself. Do unto your feet as you would unto your hands; every two, three or four weeks is sufficient.

FEET, FEET, BEAUTIFUL FEET

Not very many people have beautiful feet. Babies all have adorable feet and tweakable toes, but somewhere along the line as we reach adulthood, our feet seem to take on more character than charm. So having beautiful feet becomes a matter of creating them for yourself.

When playing Pygmalion to your feet, you have to remember how different they are from hands. While they too are working tools, they have a different kind of job and a different set of problems.

■ Toenails grow less quickly than fingernails.

■ Toenails should not be filed into a curve, especially at the sides. They should be cut straight across with a nail clipper and *never* indented at the quick—this prevents ingrowth. Ingrown nails can be helped by cutting a small V out of the nail. As the Vee grows together the nail will pull away from where it had ingrown.

■ The cuticles on toes are much tougher than those on fingers. Don't cut them, they can be pushed back with an orange stick.

■ Keep toenails short; they should *never* grow beyond the length of the toe. I suggest they be trimmed every month.

■ The sole of the foot is prone to fungus and infection. It's imperative to keep your feet clean to keep them healthy.

■ Poorly fitted shoes can cause damage to the feet. That can lead to leg trouble and even back problems.

■ Remove the top surface of calluses from feet with a scraper or pumice stone. You don't need to have velvet-soft feet—calluses are protective—but dead skin should be sloughed off regularly.

■ Never wear shoes that are too small—no matter how gorgeous or how low the sale price.

■ Alternate shoes on a daily basis. Also wear a variety of heel heights. Extremely high heels strain your calves and back.

■ Don't abandon shoes in the summer; this makes the feet spread. You don't want to have fat feet!

■ Don't walk on your toes—it's bad for the arches. If you already have fallen arches, exercise them.

■ Toenail clippers are heftier than the kind you use on your hands. Make sure you have both in your beauty-supply kit. File the top of the nails only, just to smooth them out.

■ If you are developing a corn, go to a podiatrist. Don't try to handle this problem yourself.

■ If you have a job that keeps you on your feet a lot, you should see a podiatrist and have him check out your shoes and your stockings (he may suggest support hose) as well as your feet.

THE PEDICURE

One of the greatest luxuries in the world is a pedicure—preferably a salon pedicure, since unless you are double-jointed, you will be able to relax more when someone else is hunched over your feet. A salon pedicure is usually more thorough than a home job, but home care is better than none at all, so here are some tips for your next pedicure.

Salon Pedicure

If you are wearing trousers, you'll be more comfortable if you wear knee-high hose, not panty hose. They're easier to take off and put on.

Expect a salon pedicure to last almost two hours (including drying time). Each pedicurist has a different routine: some operators use vibrators on their clients' toes; others have vibrating foot baths or foot machines; some just use a basin of warm water. The purpose of a pedicure is similar to that of the manicure—the feet will soak (they'll soak for quite a while, as the skin on the feet is tougher), cuticle will be pushed back, dead skin will be removed, your feet will be massaged (so should be your shins or calves), the toenails will be clipped and filed and then, after at least an hour's care, the polish will be applied. The polish is the least important part, as it's really just for show, while the other steps are for the good of your feet.

Whether you choose a polish color to match your fingernails or not is entirely up to you. The polish on your toes will probably last three to four weeks (although it will chip or wear on the edges if you walk in sand frequently), but it's nice to have the color in your handbag for touch-ups.

If you don't have the time to stay at the salon until your toes are completely dry, bring a pair of thong sandals. It will probably take thirty minutes or more for your toenails to dry, and I don't recommend quick-dry oils because they dull polish.

Tip the pedicurist 15 percent, whether you provide the polish or not. Check the price of a pedicure before you go—sometimes it is wildly expensive; comparison-shop. Make sure your pedicurist has a license.

Home Pedicure

Allow yourself at least an hour for your home pedicure, and this doesn't include drying time for your polish. This is the perfect activity for a rainy night, for beauty night or for a dateless Saturday when there is something you want to watch on TV (while your polish is drying—not while you are applying it). Remember that the point of the pedicure is not to apply polish to your toes, but to give your feet a reward and a health treatment.

You'll need a large mixing bowl filled with hot (over 100 degrees) water, unless you have one of those foot machines that come in various configurations. (They usually aren't too expensive and are worth the investment.) Add to your footbath some type of bubbly, soothing product—I like Vitabath. I also add a cupful of German bath salts (Epsom salts will do fine) which I buy at the drug store for less than $3 a box. Soak your feet for at least fifteen minutes; twenty is better. Read a book or watch TV. If you have a machine, flick it on for the last ten minutes so you get some good vibrations. After the soaking, use a pumice stone to remove dead skin from the sides and bottom of your feet. Do not touch corns or bunions!

Dry your feet thoroughly (wet feet breed fungus), push back cuticles with an orange stick, then clip and file toenails.

Lather on hand cream—you may like one that is thicker than a lotion. Lather and massage, working over your feet, ankles, calves and up to your knees. When you get to the knees, massage around the kneecap—not over it, because knees are too sensitive to risk dislodging that cartilage with a massage. Don't smear cream between your toes, because you should be trying to keep that area dry and fungus-free.

When you are finally ready to put on the polish, use those foam-rubber separators sold in drug and dime stores, or put tissue between your toes to separate them; otherwise you'll go nuts trying to keep your toes apart. And never give yourself a pedicure right after a manicure. This may work in the salon, where someone else is doing the work, but is bad practice for you at home. (You can, however, reverse the procedure.)

BLISTERS

Blisters are painful and ugly and should be treated properly to ward off infection. The best way to treat blisters is to prevent them. Blisters are caused by irritation—your foot rubbing against something that's resisting the skin, like your shoes or sandal strap. Feet that are damp, sweaty or wet tend to blister more easily because the skin is soft and puffy. Try some of these measures:

- If you jog or walk for sport, wear *two* pairs of socks, for absorption and for protection.
- Never buy too-tight shoes, hoping they will "stretch out." They won't!
- If a shoe is beginning to rub and you know a blister is coming, apply baby powder and use a Band-Aid at the first hint of trouble. Change Band-Aids often, as they can get rubbed, sweaty and dirty in no time at all.
- Do not pop blisters without following up with careful attention. Clean a needle with alcohol before inserting into the blister. Clean blisters well, expose to fresh air for a few minutes, then open with a sterile needle, wash with disinfectant (even if it burns) and protect with a padded bandage or sterile piece of gauze and Band-Aid. (Do not sterilize the needle by lighting a match to the tip—this will get carbon on the needle and into your foot. Instead, thread the needle, then drop it into boiling water while still holding the thread in your hand.)
- Take pressure off a blister by cutting out a hole in a gauze or moleskin pad to build up the area surrounding it.

FOOT DOCTORS

Just to show you the importance of your feet, you should know that there are several different doctors (some medical doctors or M.D.s, others licensed by the state in which they practice) who deal with foot problems, and then there are other specialists as well.

Orthopedic surgeon: a bone specialist. If your feet need to be operated on, he's your man. He will probably take only referral patients—those sent to him (or her) from other specialists.

Podiatrist: a foot specialist who is not an M.D., but who is expert at handling corns, blisters and assorted foot problems.

Reflexogist: not an M.D. He or she believes that every part of the body has a home base somewhere in the foot and that foot "massage" of the pressure points can cure health problems in other areas. Can be painful.

Chiropractor: not an M.D., but licensed by the state and called "Doctor." He or she gives medical treatment focused more on the back and legs than the feet, but often your feet cause problems in these other areas.

FOOT TIPS

■ Keep feet as dry as possible at all times. Foot powder (without starch) helps in this area.

■ If you have pain when you walk, consult a doctor.

■ Don't expect a pair of shoes to *get* comfortable. You will have a good deal of pain and may never "break them in." You will be broken instead. If they aren't comfortable when you buy them, forget them, no matter how gorgeous.

■ Always try each shoe. Don't buy a pair you didn't try on.

■ If your feet are cold at night, wear bed socks to bed.

■ If you cannot afford regular pedicures, have one at the beginning of the summer season and one at the end.

■ Wear proper shoes for the occasion, including sports and walking.

■ Don't buy a size 6 shoe if the 6½ really feels more comfortable just because you have always worn size 6 in the past. A shoe from manufacturer "A" may not run the same size as a shoe from manufacturer "B." Shoes vary, and a 6½ B in black may not feel exactly like the 6½ B in brown.

CONTEMPLATING YOUR FEET

I once suggested to a client that she come in for a pedicure as a special treat to herself. "Oh, no," she said, "my feet are the worst! I'd be too embarrassed."

Believe me, the pedicurist has seen less beautiful feet than yours. She's there to help you, and you really need the help so don't be embarrassed. A pedicure is important because it keeps the toenails from rubbing against your shoes and causing swelling in your feet. You need to have dead skin eliminated regularly and to prevent callus buildup. There are real health benefits to a pedicure. *And,* having a pedicure is like wearing silk underwear—you feel beautiful from top to bottom. You're worth it!

I like to take a little time each morning right after I wake up to lie in bed to do some foot exercises. This is a bit like meditation and gives you a nice peaceful feeling first thing in the day.

1. Wake Up Toes. Sit up in bed with toes straight out and point, then hold and count to 10, ten times. Then flex and hold, count to 10 and release. Repeat ten times also.
2. Ankle Circles. While lying in bed, raise one leg at a time and fully rotate at the ankle. Repeat ten times, then alternate legs.
3. Rise and Shine. Now out of bed and onto your phone book. Stand on top of the phone book (It should be at least two inches thick) and place your feet at the edge so your toes can hang over. Then curl your toes in. Repeat ten times.

These few minutes of foot time will help you start your day better. You can then begin your regular exercise program (I do), or proceed to the shower to get going on your day. A few minutes for yourself (and your feet) will pace your day, and start you off on the, uh, right foot.

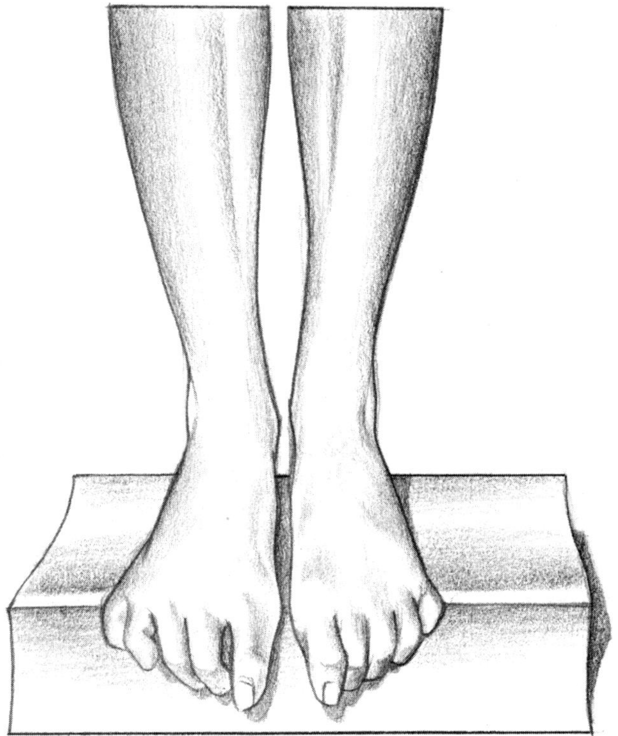

Squeeze!

Eight

Makeup

MAKING MAGIC

Makeup *is* magic. It turns a plain girl into a glorious woman; it makes a bare face sparkle with interesting facets. It can't do *everything*, but when it's used with finesse and know-how, look out, world—the not-so-natural beauties are about to make their mark!

Once you have clear, smooth skin and hair that glistens in the sun, you will find makeup the finishing touch to a more beautiful you. If you have yet to perfect the essentials, take your time; there's no reason to worsen a skin condition by trying to hide it under a pound of Pancake. Get the guidance you need to clear your complexion, *then* learn the makeup tricks that will enhance your basics. If your problems are more severe than the usual blemishes that plague all of us, perhaps you need to look ahead to Chapter Nine.

Putting on makeup should be a relaxing, pleasant experience because you are taking the time to do something positive for yourself. Even when you're under the weather, don't you feel better after you've put some makeup on? Enhancing your looks should be considered an art. We all have our quick little makeup tricks, and every woman should know how to put on a five-minute face (see page 143), but your daily routine should be rewarding and enjoyable, well worth the ten to twenty minutes of your time it takes.

Because so much money is spent annually on makeup, cosmetics have become a multi-billion-dollar business. The competition for your dollars is keen, so before you fall sway to advertising, salespeople or a pretty packaging, here are some overall rules to guide you:

- Except for foundation and blush, all makeup products are pretty much the same, and you can choose whatever brand or price range you want on the basis of color and texture preferences.
- Before you buy a new shade of lipstick or eye shadow, look around. Often all the

fashion lines come out with similar colors, so you may be able to find what you want in a less expensive version.

■ Buying and using makeup is an acquired skill. Don't expect something new to look good on first application. It's like playing the piano—practice counts!

■ Usually, the salesperson at the department-store makeup counter is an employee of the cosmetic company, not the store—something most people don't know. She has been trained exclusively with the cosmetics of the company she works for, and her job is to sell you something from that line—*not* to tell you what is the best thing for your look.

■ Dime-store brands don't usually have fashion colors, so if you want the latest looks, check out the department stores. In the long run, you may actually save money by paying department-store prices, since you'll be getting the colors you want with the first purchase.

■ Remember, don't judge how a product will look on you by how it looks on a model. Pictures are retouched, shot from tricky angles and lit to make the models look better than Wonder Woman.

If you panic when you shop for makeup, or need some direction, make some decisions before you set out. Perhaps a small boutique or a private salon is better for you than a huge store. Never buy makeup on a whim unless you are prepared to write it off and take the loss. Research what you are looking for and test a few brands on your hand. Testing is always free. The search should be fun. Remember, since skin-care products within one line are formulated to work together, it's better to use one brand for your entire care program. But when it comes to makeup, you can use several different brands if you like. It may be easier to buy all your cosmetics in one stop, but it is not imperative. Don't ever let anyone tell you that one product won't work, or look right, unless you use others in the line. When you are picking colors, check out the fashions and pictures in magazines and size up your own look. Some colors become dated quickly, and you can end up with a nice makeup in *unfashionable* shades if you are not careful.

Always allow a makeup artist to do your face when you are trying something new. You'll pick up tricks from a pro, and if you don't like the end result, you can always wash your face. (It's not like having your hair cut and waiting months for it to grow out.) But be sure to tell the makeup artist what you didn't like and why. Makeup artists who represent major lines and give in-store demonstrations usually do so for free; if the demonstrator asks before the session that you commit yourself to buying some of her products, move to another counter. If you don't mind being made up in front of strangers, this is a good way to experiment with no obligation to buy. If you go to a small salon, like ours, ask if it does complimentary makeup sessions. You should never feel pressured to buy.

If you are influenced by a picture in a magazine, take some time to analyze it. Is the product something you can use, or are you being sold by romance and glamour? I think it's better to save your money to buy three good products rather than to buy ten less expensive "hot" items you may use once or twice, only to discover they are just not for you.

If you decide to go to a makeup artist, be sure your skin is absolutely clean. This way you will be able to see the true color of the makeup on your skin. When trying to decide between two similar colors of shadow, place a little on the inside of your wrist to test the true shade; two brown shadows may appear to be the exact same shade when you see them in the case, but are really different when applied to the skin. We all make mistakes with makeup, but after some trial and error you should be able to keep these to a minimum. The person who rushes out to buy all new cosmetics every spring and fall, or is constantly changing her look, is seeking a satisfaction she will never find in a package. Know who you are and what your look is before you go shopping for the magic.

FINDING YOUR TYPE

The key to looking your best is finding the right beauty approach for your personality and lifestyle. You need to create your own look, not copy someone else's. It's okay to borrow a little here and a little there, but you'll never build confidence until you know what is right for *you* and you alone.

One of the best ways to find your beauty type is to experiment. Try several different styles and ask a friend to take a series of instant pictures. Look at yourself objectively, then decide which look suits you. Among the women I see, there are a couple of perennially popular looks.

Sophisticated. The sophisticated look is a classic, plus. Hair, clothes, nails and makeup are sharp and up-to-date. While the makeup doesn't change dramatically, the clothes and accessories are always *au courant;* hair is always sleek, perfect and neat. Makeup colors are bright and strong.

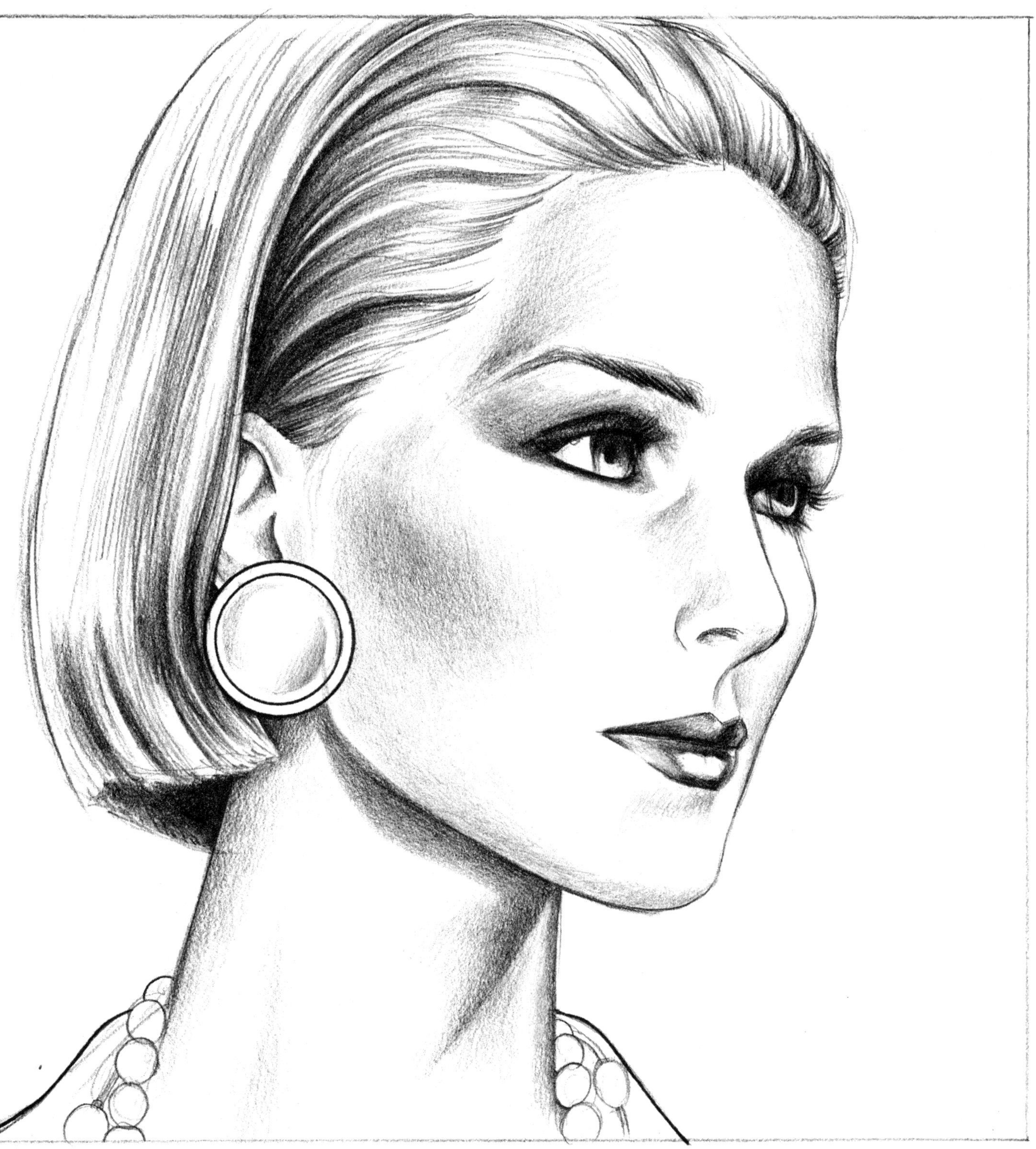

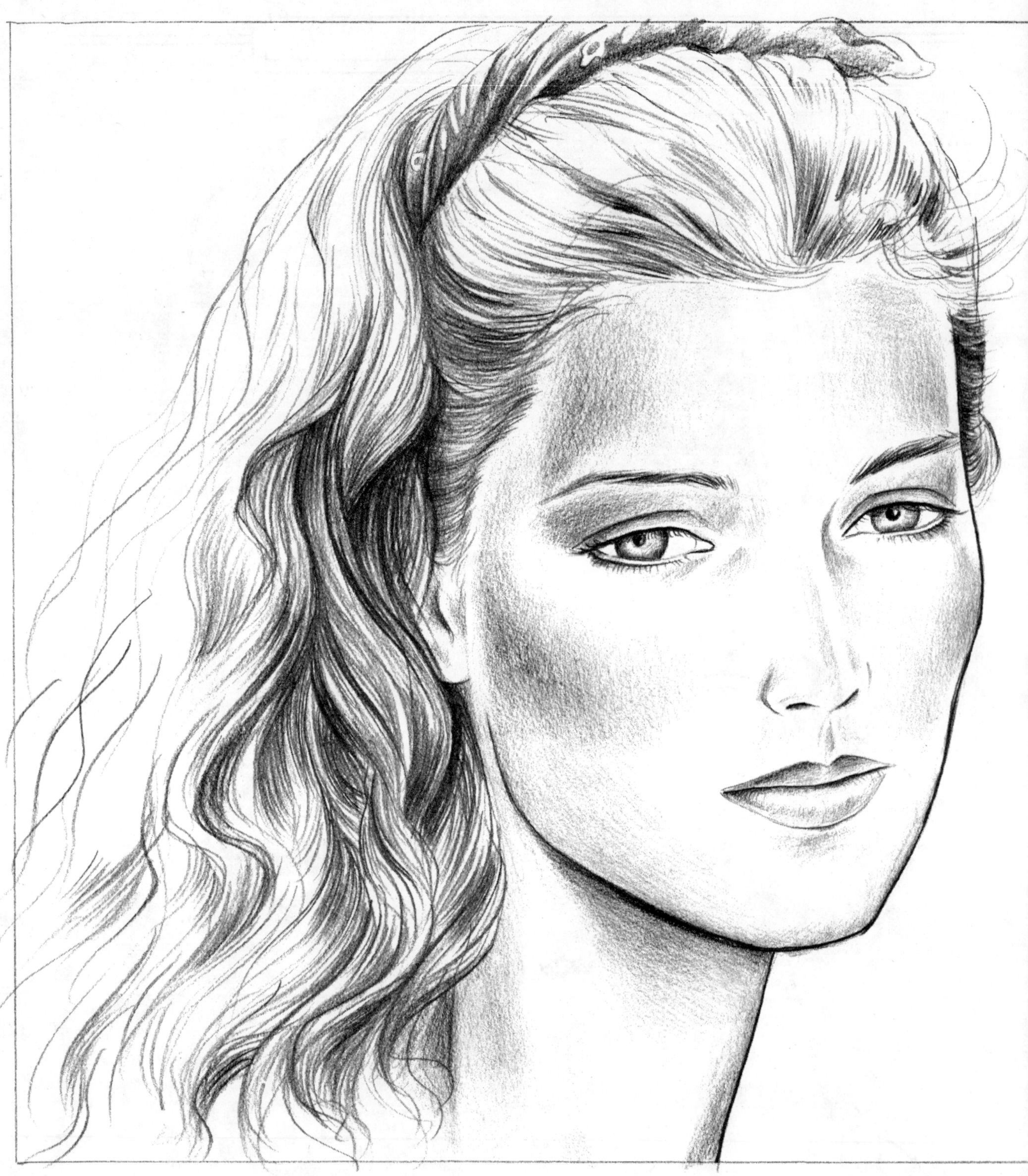

Outdoorsy. The outdoorsy type is the clean, lean and healthy look. The color in her cheeks is natural, not blush. The glow she has is from good circulation. There's nothing studied about this look. Mascara and lip gloss are her maximum beauty touches.

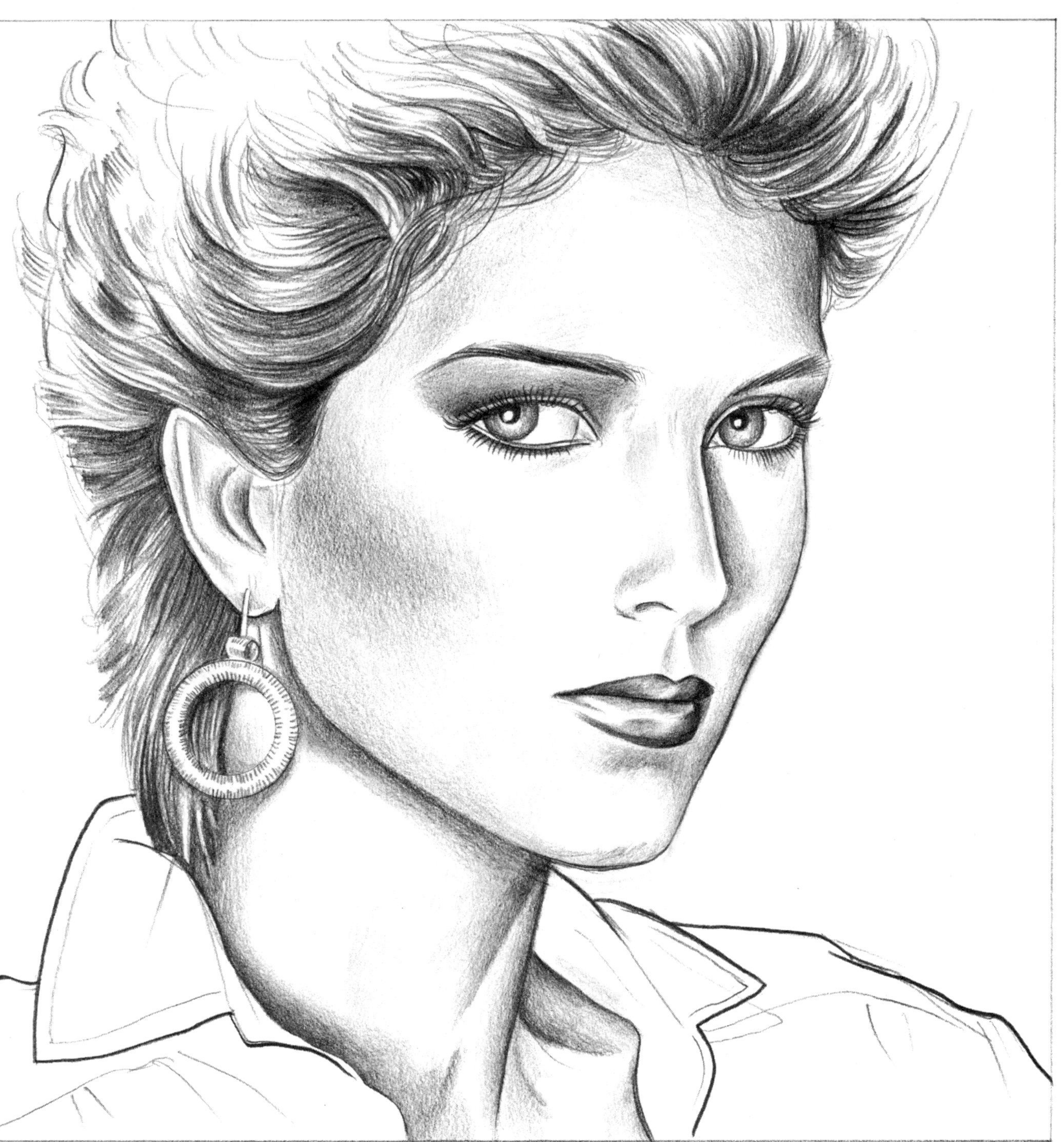

Natural. The natural look is nothing like the outdoorsy look, believe it or not. While it may sound like a contradiction in terms, it takes a good bit of makeup for many people to look "natural." Selecting muted tones (brown-based colors) can help create this effect. You can give yourself the natural look, but you cannot achieve the outdoorsy look without living the life. If you decide to go natural, the key to success is blend, blend, blend all your cosmetics, so no one can see where one begins and the other ends.

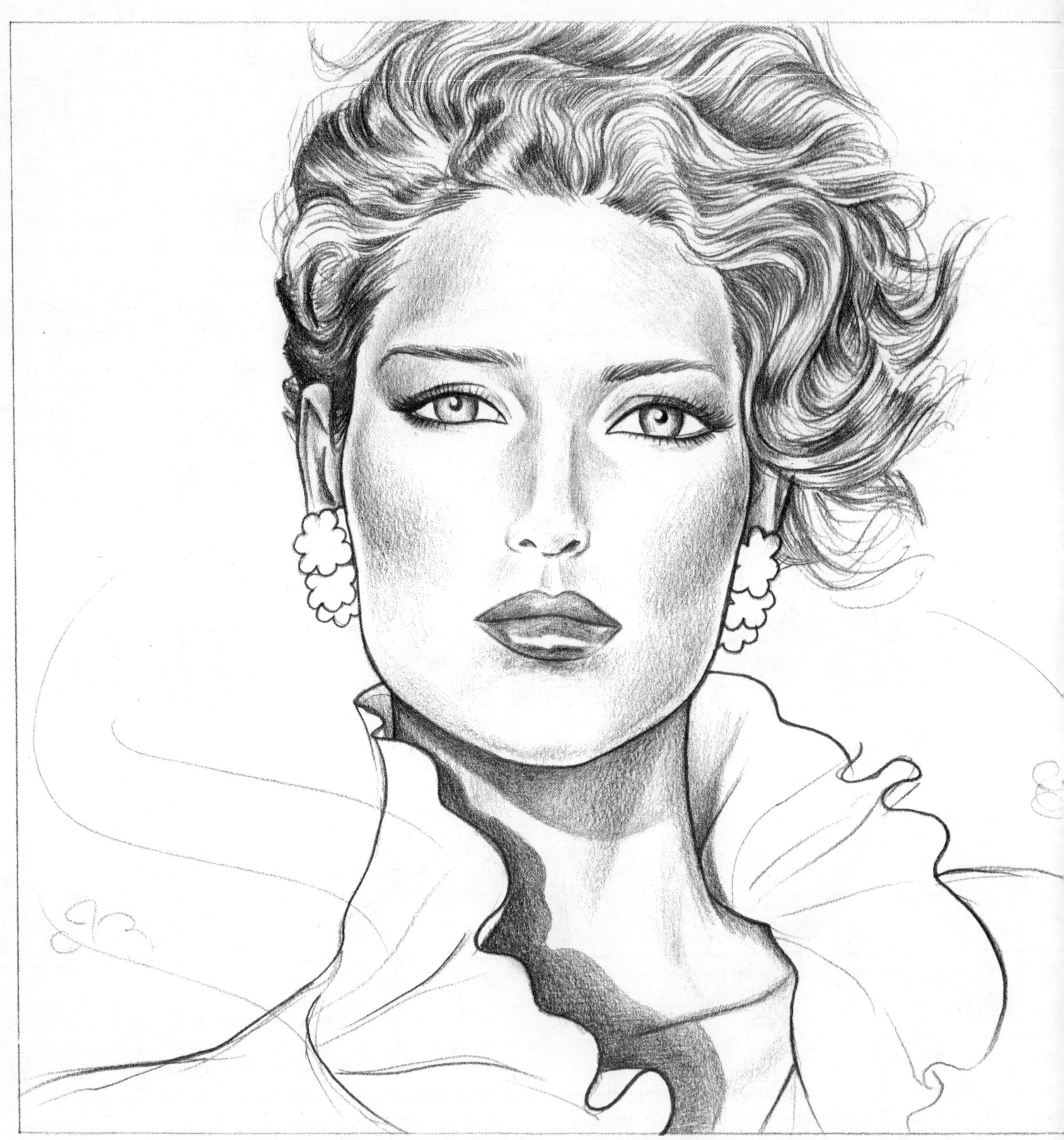

Feminine. The feminine look is soft and subtle. It takes more makeup than the natural look—pretty colors and balanced tones. The feminine look requires pastel or floral shades all in the same color family, nothing too bright. Short curls and a very feminine floral fragrance go with this look.

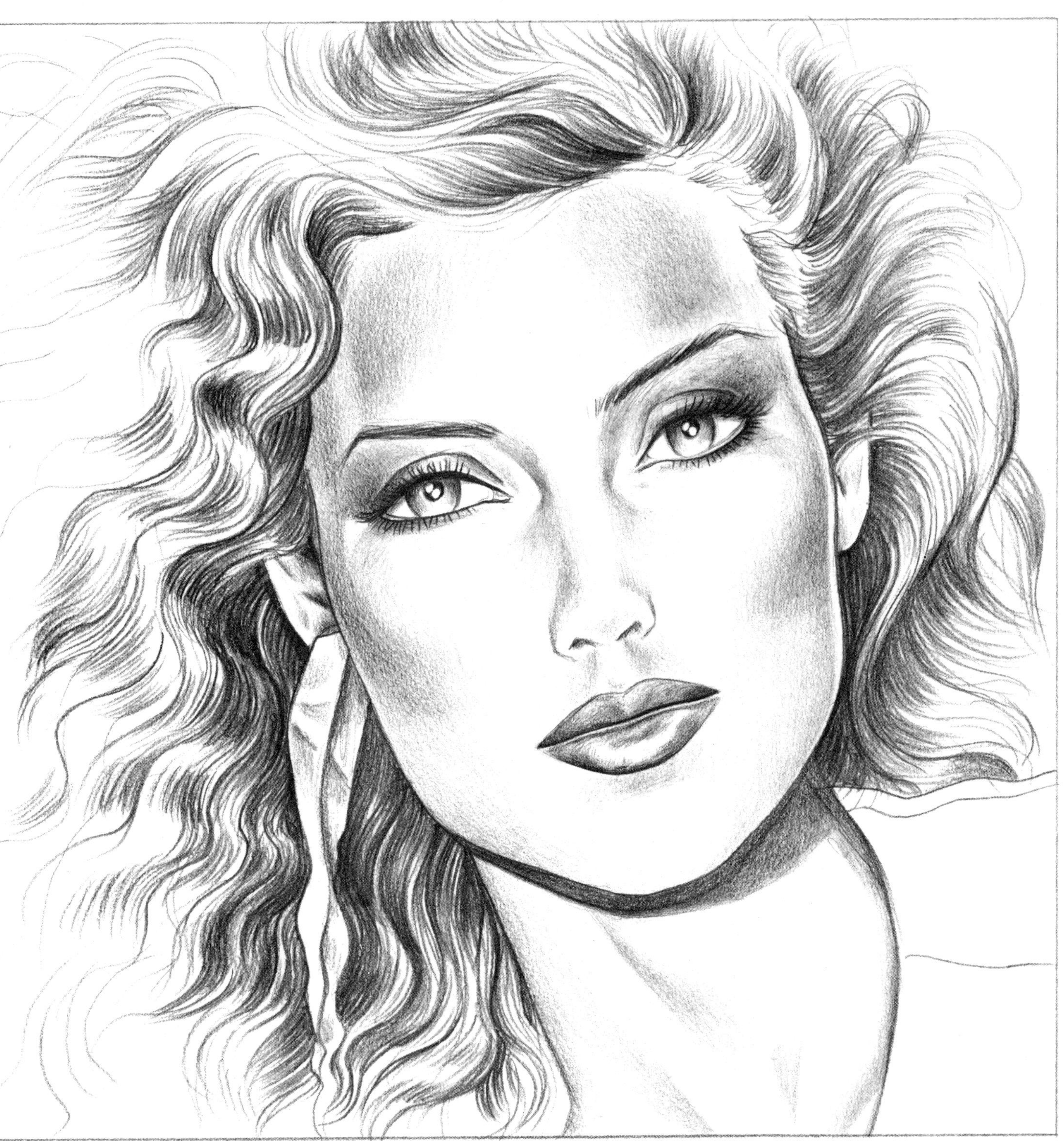

Sultry. Sultry is actually more an attitude than a look, but this type of woman exudes it —her makeup is flirty and coquettish, she aims to look sexy. (Usually a pouty mouth is part of the look.) Emphasis is on the eyes or the mouth. The sultry woman knows what her best feature is and how to make it look exceptional.

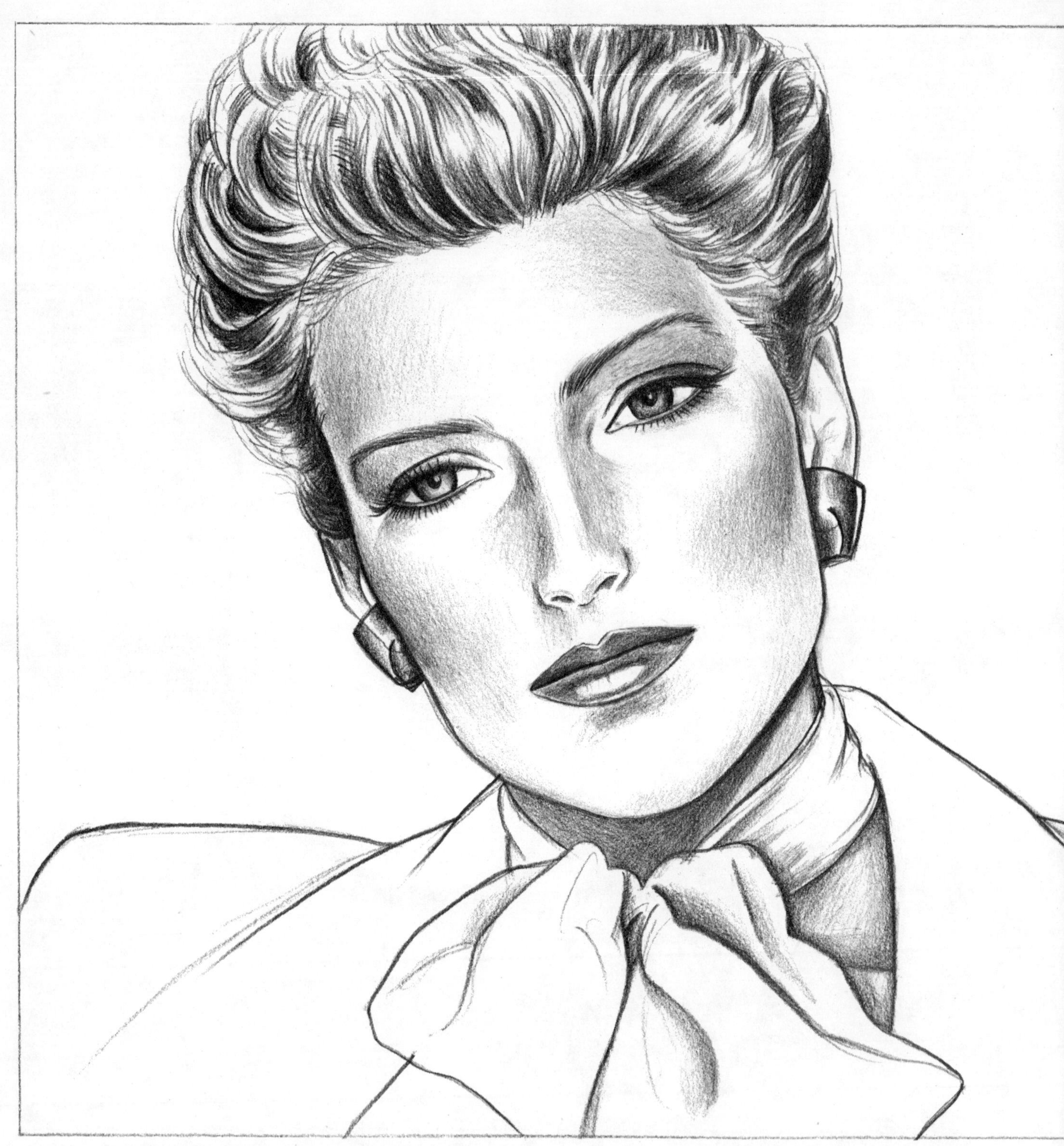

Managerial. Neat is the operative word here. Usually it's a toned-down, tightened-up version of the woman's own look, made suitable for the corporate world of dressing for success. The look says attractive, not threatening. No fragrance evident.

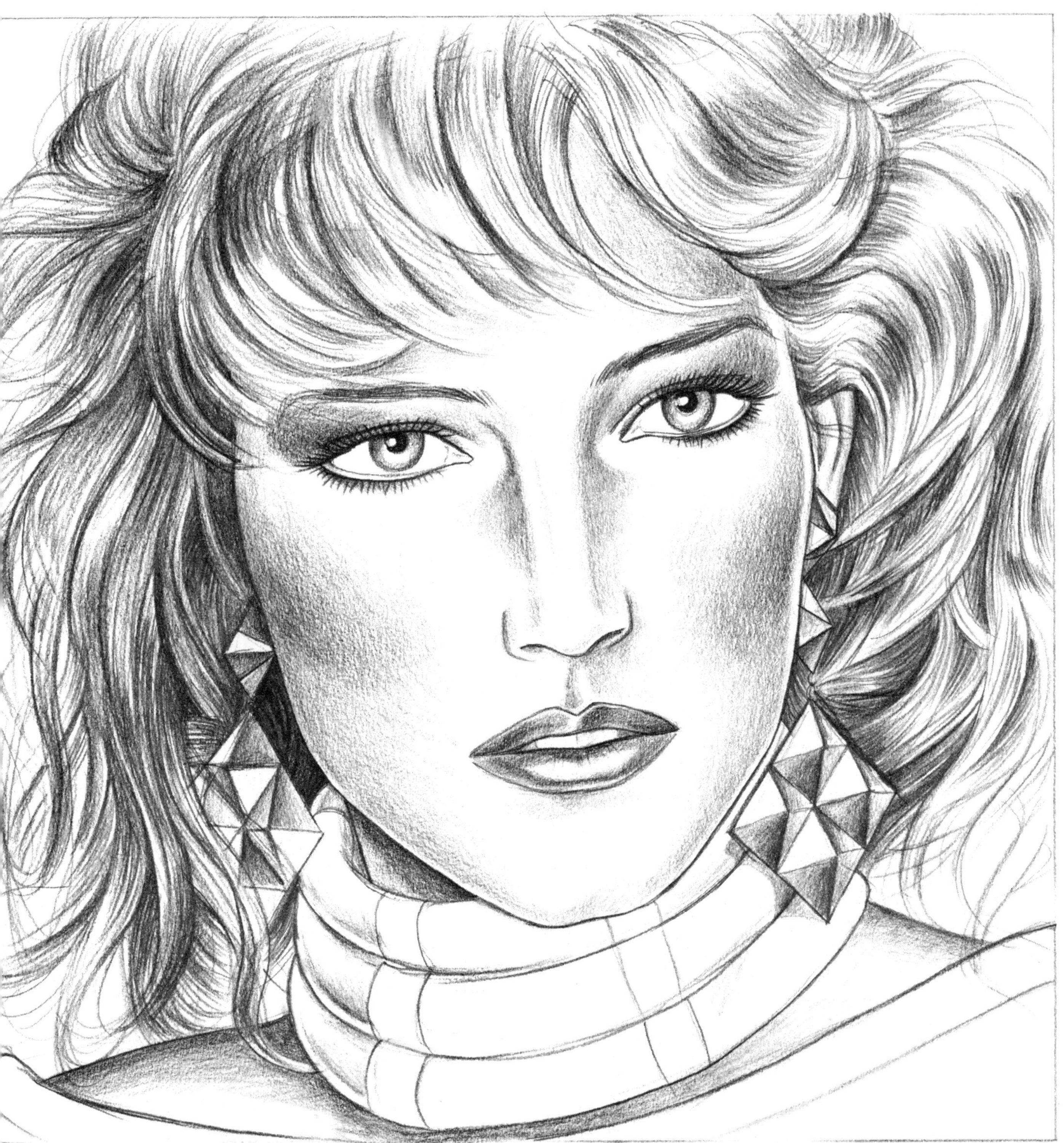

Hip. She looks tousled yet somehow fashionable and chic. It takes time to look studied/messy, because you aren't going out in the world barefaced or without a hairstyle. Colors are apparent but not strident. The casualness is there, but it's worked on, honed to perfection.

Choosing the look for you will depend on a few variables:

1. Are there clothing and fashion restrictions where you work? Are some looks totally unsuitable?
2. Do your peers all look a certain way?
3. What makes you feel most comfortable?
4. Do you have a fantasy vision of yourself that you long to achieve?
5. Would you like to look better but don't know where to start?
6. Do your parents influence your self-image? Would you like to look a certain way but find it unacceptable for school or home?
7. Do you like a certain look but lack the technical know-how to achieve it?
8. Do you like a certain look but lack the right personality to pull it off? Remember, every look suggests a type of behavior.

COLOR ME BEAUTIFUL

Today many people are having their colors done, which can be fun. However, as the colors are being draped around you, remember that the makeup you are wearing at the time will influence what looks best. Many colors that don't seem becoming could look good on you if your makeup were altered accordingly. (For example, if you like hot pink but are afraid to wear it: apply a bright pink lipstick and bright pink rouge, and the hot pink outfit will probably be super.) But clothes should not "wear you"—you should not appear overpowered by your attire.

Before making up each day, decide what you will be wearing so that you can choose appropriate colors. I am always rushing in the morning, so every night I pull out something to wear and line up my eye shadows and lipstick so I won't have to make frenzied decisions.

THE MAKE-OVER

Susannah was thirty-four when she came to see me. She had been a student until she was thirty, earning a Ph.D. in theater arts, then won a Fulbright to study theater abroad. She lived on a small stipend and had no money for clothes or cosmetics. Besides, in her circle, no makeup and blue jeans were the rule.

Over the last three years Susannah had been writing and directing plays, again as a starving beginner. Then suddenly, she had a hit. Overnight she was being asked to meet important people, see agents and actors and join glittering theatrical parties. She needed a new look, but she didn't even have an old one. She had never even applied makeup and had no idea what was "right" for her.

She had her hair styled and her "mus-

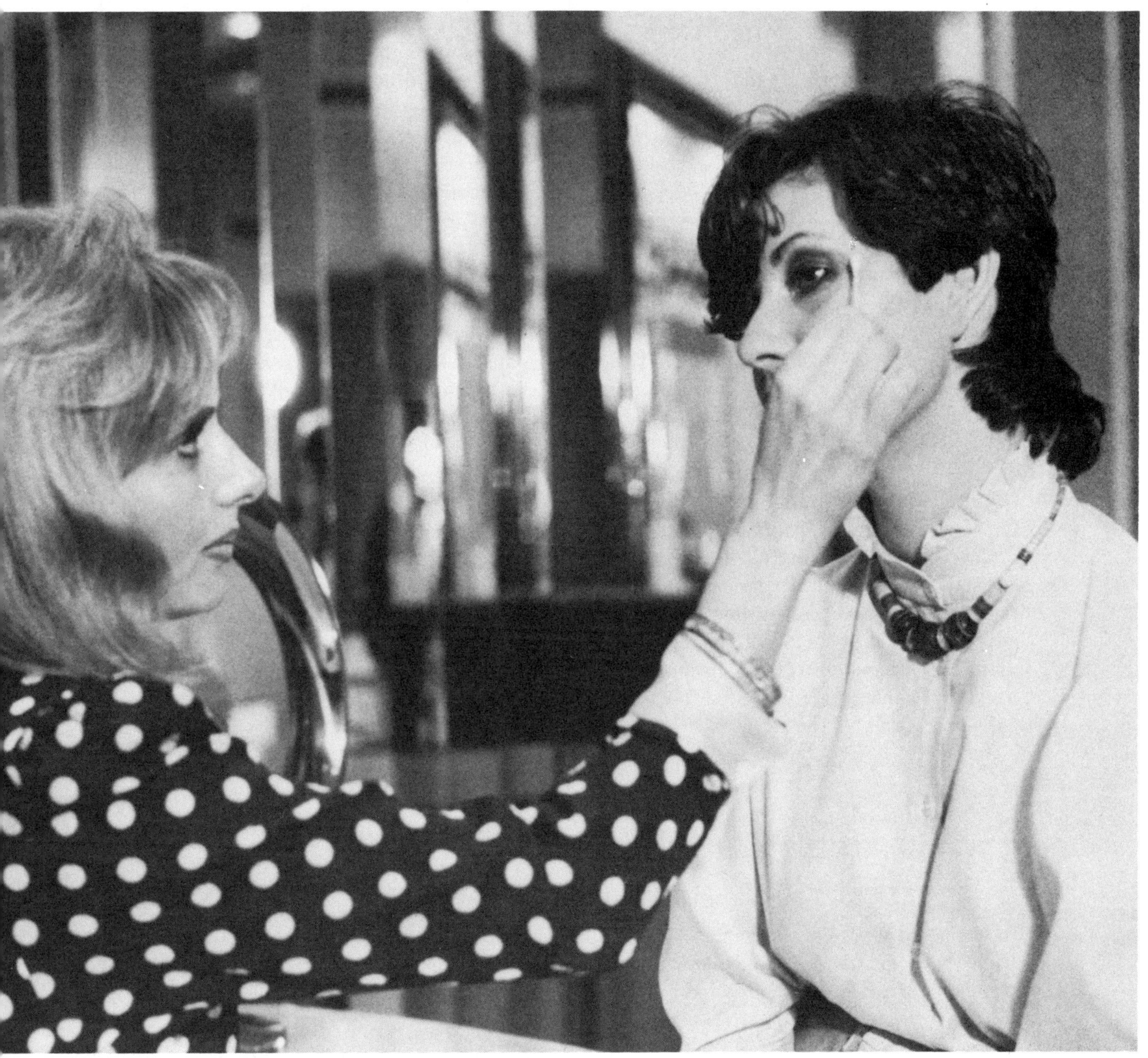

In the salon, helping a client discover a new look

tache" waxed and received treatment for her oily skin. She learned to apply makeup and develop her own style. It took about a month to turn her into a swan. Now she laughs at old pictures of herself.

At twenty-two, Jessica was excited about interviewing for her first job. To her dismay, she found herself in reception areas with other women who were also interviewing who looked far more sophisticated. Although she had liked her waist-length blond hair and natural makeup look (her mom and boyfriend liked it too), she realized that if she was going to compete in the business world, she had better do something to spruce up her image. She got new makeup, concentrating on her eyes, had her hair trimmed and splurged on a well-tailored but feminine interview suit. Now she's an account exec.

Bored with her same old "safe" appearance, Clara saved up her money and went to the fanciest hairstylist in town, then had an appointment with his makeup artist. She told them only that she was tired of looking ordinary and wanted to look bold and sexy. They could do whatever they wanted—transformation was the name of the game. A haircut, a perm and new makeup, and Clara also *felt* different—which made her *act* differently. She enjoyed her new look so much that she began to rethink her whole self-image and decided she could do far better with her life and career. This newfound determination enabled her to forge ahead to realize what she had thought was only a fantasy.

At age twenty-one, my friend Lacey was pursuing a modeling career in New York City. Although she was one of the more beautiful hopefuls, she rarely got a booking. Finally, she asked why. The answer surprised her: she didn't look as if she *needed* a job. Not that she should have looked disheveled or poverty-stricken—but wearing diamond earrings and designer silks to interviews gave the impression she was more the social gadabout than a hardworking, dependable person. She learned to tone down her look, wearing well-cut but modest clothes with a minimum of adornment, and found that her beauty, not her lifestyle, shone through.

PICKING COSMETICS

Cosmetics are not all created equal, but often there is little difference between them—except for price. How should you pick one from another? I choose my cosmetics by these criteria:

1. Ingredients. Read the label. The label will tell you exactly (almost exactly) what's in the product, and in what proportions. The ingredients are listed in descending order of amounts included. If you are buying a collagen makeup but collagen is listed last, you'll know there isn't too much in there.

2. Price. Remember, always go for a middle-of-the-road price range—not too inexpensive, not too expensive. Buy what you can afford; don't go without lunch to have the money to pay for the most expensive product out there. But if you see a pretty item that makes you feel good and still allows you to feed your piggy bank and you really want it,

go ahead and treat yourself. The costs of the advertising, the fancy models, the retouched picture and the packaging all are absorbed in the price. A product from a modest firm can be as good as one from one of the big houses—you just tend to trust the big houses because you are familiar with their names. And that is a function of The Big Sell.

3. Usability. I don't buy fad makeup, because I like classic good looks for all women. But if change excites you, buy less expensive items so you can toss them out when they go out of style.

Foundation

Foundation is the most important part of your makeup wardrobe, because it sets the base for the rest of your cosmetics and your whole look. Your foundation must be good for both your skin and your fashion statement.

■ Never test a foundation on your hand. The skin on your hand is usually a different color from the skin on your face. Try instead a test area under your jaw. The foundation color must blend with your neck or you'll have a line, which is the first makeup no-no. *Nothing* is worse than a big stripe across your neck!

■ Don't judge a color by what it looks like in the bottle. You must try it on. Refuse to buy a product you can't sample free.

■ Always have a darker shade to mix with your regular one when you want a bit of summer color. Mix it in the palm of your hand so you can control the shade.

Before you buy your base, be sure you know your skin type (see page 32), and don't let anyone change your mind.

■ There are several types of foundation on the market:

Oil-free: has no oil in it at all and is good for oily skin or acne. It would be too drying for dry or even normal skin. Two coats can be applied for maximum coverage.

Water-base: may have some oils in it, and is good for oily or normal skin or people who don't need much coverage. You can always apply two coats of base for heavier coverage.

Moisture-base: for dry skin, has emollients to give skin a glowing finish.

Oil-base: for very dry skin, usually for older women.

Cream-base: whipped or in compact form, usually too heavy for young skin; good for mature skin or for people appearing on television, since it gives heavy coverage.

Tinted moisturizer: a possible substitute for base, but I don't recommend it because you shouldn't put moisturizer everywhere you need to put a foundation. And in order to accommodate the color, the moisturizer is not as good as it should be.

■ Never apply foundation with the fingertips. Use a clean makeup sponge instead.

■ Never apply foundation over old makeup. Apply to clean skin only.

■ Buy makeup without fragrance in it to avoid irritation and discoloration—the fragrance can react with the sun to cause brown spots on your skin.

■ If your skin *feels* heavy, or as if it were suffocating, your foundation is too heavy. Foundation should sit lightly on *top* of skin, not be pressed into it. It will help to use a sponge to apply your foundation.

■ Because foundation goes directly next to your skin, buy one carefully, and buy the best you can afford, because it is, in fact, more a part of your skin-care routine than your makeup ritual.

■ If you use liquid foundation, replace the cap immediately after using—the liquid can dry up or get crusty.

Eye Shadow

There are so many different eye shadows in so many different formulas that you will have to experiment to find the best ones for you. If your look is classical or businesslike, your eye shadow probably will not change much over the years, although you should have a night version for special occasions. If you are in a more sophisticated fashion mode, you may vary your fashion statement by changing your eyeshadow colors without altering any other aspect of your makeup.

■ Always put cream foundation on your lid under the brow and under eyes before applying shadow. This way you get the true color of the shadow and much longer-lasting wear.

■ Experimenting with makeup is natural and should be fun—especially experimenting with eye shadows, because there are myriad possibilities. Just never go out of the house until you have perfected a look. If you can't apply the product perfectly, don't use it! Practice does make a world of difference.

■ If you're unhappy with a shadow, try it in many ways before you discard it. (Then don't give it away, throw it away if it flunks.) A shadow might work as an eyeliner or, if the color is too bright, try it just on the outside corner of the lid. Lots of shadows can be used wet or dry. Wet ones are less likely to flake—especially important to people who wear contact lenses.

■ Wet shadows are usually darker than powder shadows and stay on longer.

■ Sticks and creams often look tempting, but they may not stay on as well and may smear as the oils in the product disperse.

■ Glimmers and shimmers (loose powdered shadows that come in a small pot) are hard to work with. Be sure to flick excess off the brush before you apply, or try a sponge-tip applicator. Gold dust in your eye will not be welcome. But don't be afraid to use it. It's fun for evenings or special occasions.

■ Pressed cake eye shadow is best for most people, and easiest to apply. Some pearl gives the shadow a softer consistency so it is easier to blend. Liquid eyeliner has not been in style for over a decade, but eyeliners in pencil form are popular. Try using a bright shadow as a liner. I love to do this.

■ Always smudge eyeliner. If you line top and bottom, make sure they meet at outside corner. Then smudge outward.

■ Do not use a marking pen for an eyeliner!

■ Use cotton swabs or sponge tips for smudging eyeliner. If you insist on using your fingertips, make sure your hands are clean. Don't worry about drawing a perfect line; the swab or sponge tip will work wonders for cleaning up and perfecting lines.

■ As you experiment with eyeliner pencils, you'll notice that different brands spread differently. When lining the eyes, you shouldn't have to push the skin around to get the color on. Always test eyeliner pencils on the hand to be sure they will flow easily on the eyelids. If not, return them!

Powder

There are two types of powders: face powder, shaded to match your skin tone or flatter it slightly, and colored powders, usually known as blush-ons, that come in pink, peach, orange, plum and brown shades for contouring cheeks and hollows. I think powder makes skin look dry, unhealthy and unnatural. You want your skin to have a healthy-looking glow. If you hate your shiny nose, limit powder to that area. Apply with a piece of cotton, or mix a little with your foundation on your makeup sponge.

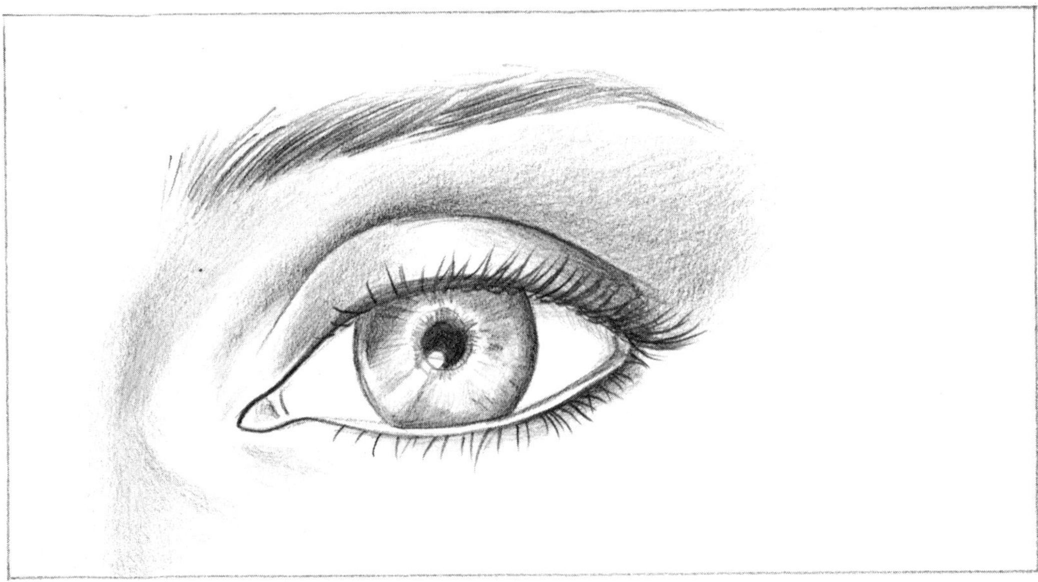

Soft, subtle shadowing for day/office

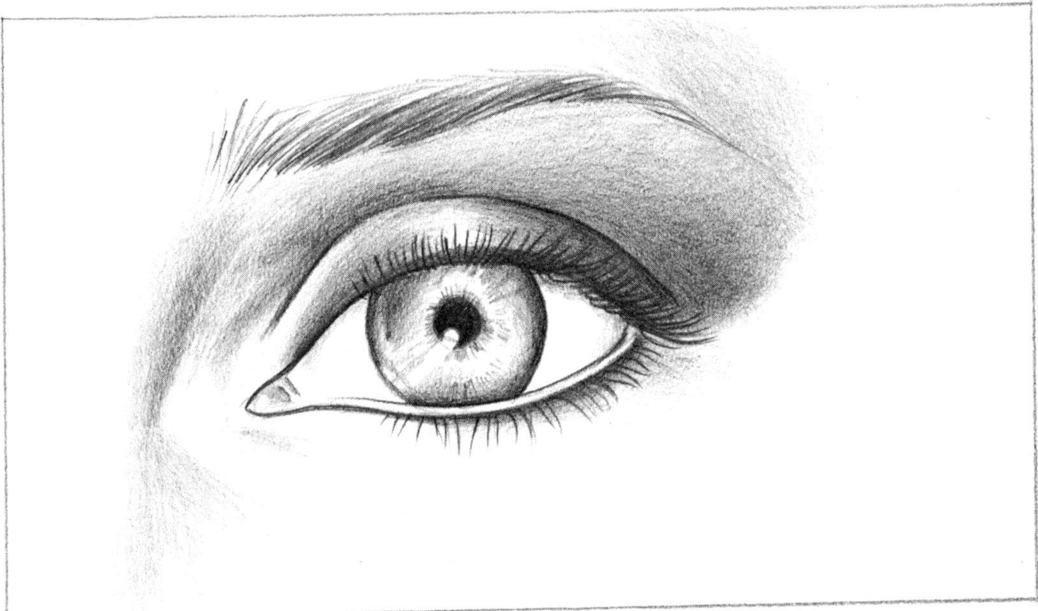

The same shadow, applied more intensely in crease and outside corner for a dramatic evening look

Rouge

Rouge may be a powder blush or a cream-base or even a gel, although gels are harder to control and I don't recommend them. They also come in stick and tube form and pencils, as well. Personally, I don't favor powder blush either. Powder rouge gets into your pores, mixes with the oils in your skin and causes clogging. Many times when I analyze skin in the salon, I am able to tell who uses powder blush and who doesn't just by the blackheads on the top of the cheeks or blush-colored dots in the pores. The resins that keep the blush together in its case get onto the brush you use to apply it. The brush

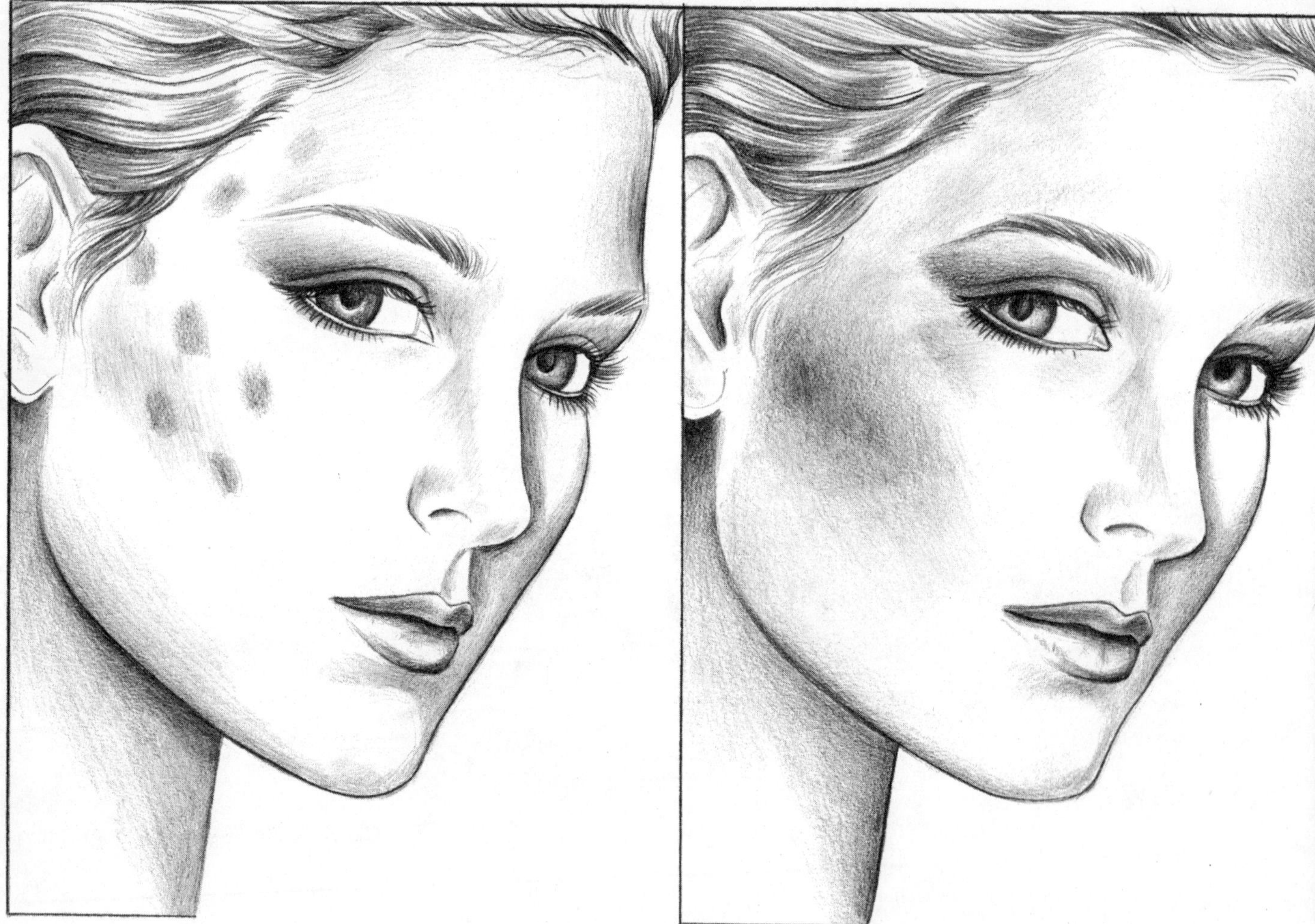

Apply rouge to cheekbone and temple

Blend well across cheek and into hairline

picks up bacteria from your skin, which are then transferred onto the blush itself each time you sweep the brush over it. This is what clogs your pores and causes problems such as blackheads and even blemishes.

■ Use a sponge to apply and blend cream rouges.

■ Where you put the rouge depends on your face shape, but always blend across the cheekbones into the hairline—don't stop short.

■ Don't go too far into the face or too close to the eye, or your face will look swollen or sunburned.

■ You should *never* see where rouge starts or stops. I suggest starting at the spot on your cheekbone directly below the pupil of your eye and blending up into the hairline.

■ One rouge product is enough; you do not need to layer colors or apply several different shades one on top of another except for special evenings or photography sessions.

■ Apply rouge, blend well with sponge, then reapply to areas that need more color and pat with sponge.

■ If you are contouring, use two products in the same color family. Be careful not to create dirty brown smudges on your face that you think pass for hollows but are really just silly-looking.

■ Remember, your makeup should look just as good close up as it does across the room.

Lipstick

Even if you are the natural type, you still need to wear lipstick because it protects your lips. The average person should have a three-color basic lipstick wardrobe—two daytime colors, one sportier than the other, and one nighttime shade.

■ Lipstick is difficult to judge on yourself; get some opinions. Remember, a lipstick color that looks great on your friend may not go with your own skin coloring.

■ To judge a lipstick, look at it on a completely made-up face; don't look just at your lips. Look at yourself from at least one foot away in order to judge the total effect.

■ Don't match lips to nails or clothes. Choose what is flattering to you. The wrong lip color can ruin an otherwise perfect makeup job.

■ Give yourself some time to get used to yourself in lipstick.

■ Put foundation on your lips before applying lipstick; this will help the lipstick stay on. Be sure there is no gap between your foundation and your lipstick.

■ Outline your lips with a lip pencil. The pencil may match the lipstick, may be brownish to coordinate with a pale shade of gloss or lipstick or may be slightly jazzier than the lipstick. These three choices depend on the look you seek.

■ If your lips need their shape enhanced, experiment a little with the lining pencil. Make a full lip thinner by drawing a line just inside your natural lip line or a thin lip more sensual by penciling just on the *out*side of your natural line. Your lipstick should *balance* your eye makeup, not overpower it. If you select a light liner pencil it will enlarge the lip line.

■ If you don't like the look of lipstick, use a lip-lining pencil, and apply a pale frosted or natural gloss.

■ Apply lipstick with a lip brush for greater control and longer staying power.

■ Put gloss on top of your lipstick, not Vaseline.

■ Take off lipstick when you remove your makeup and clean the area well or you may

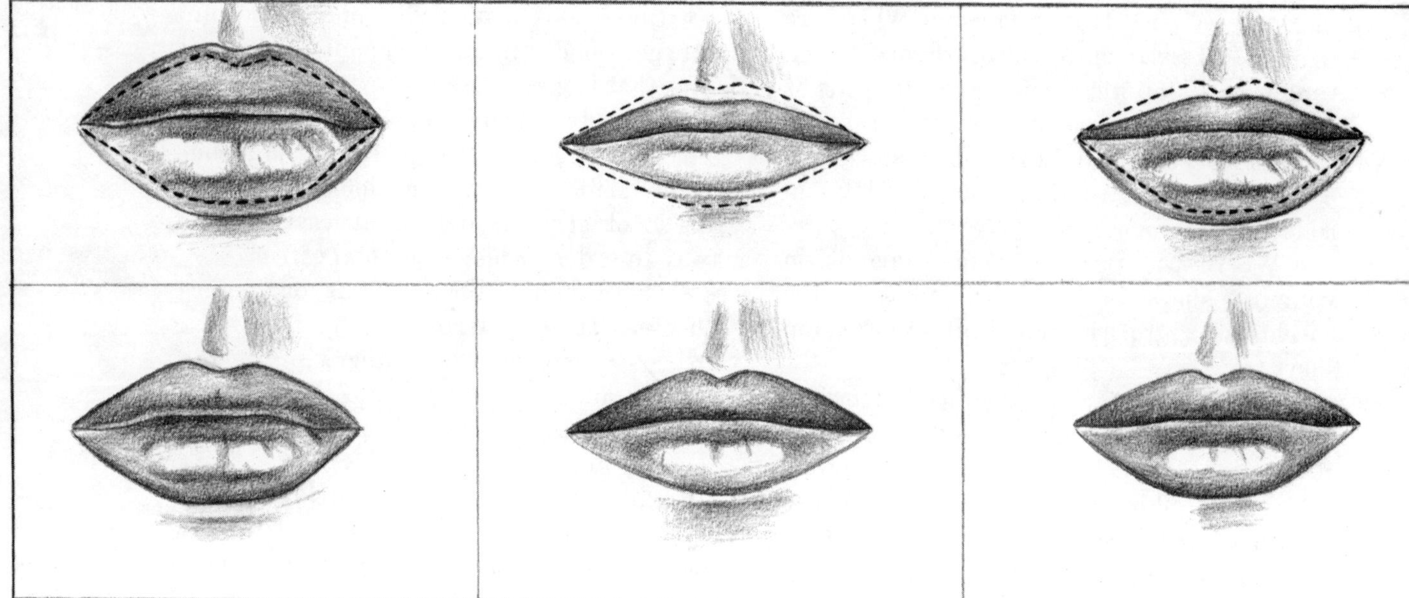

Concealing too-full lips *Enhancing thin lips* *Balancing uneven lips*

develop blackheads around your lips from clogged pores.

■ Too-small lips can be enlarged with pale lip color. For example, if the bottom lip is much thinner than the top, use a lighter lipstick for the bottom lip. Of course the tone should be similar to the top. The reverse works too. If you want to make a lip smaller, select a darker color.

Mascara

I've never had very good eyelashes—mine are blond and not especially thick—so I've always been a slave to mascara. I used to use it on both upper and lower lashes to make my eyes look bigger, but the lower lashes always smudged. The effect was wilting raccoon. One day I didn't put the mascara on the bottom. I got several compliments. So there's a lot of room for maneuvering to find what's best for you.

■ Apply mascara in three sections—inside lashes toward the nose, middle lashes straight out and outside lashes toward the hairline. This defines the whole eye and frames it properly.

■ Begin the mascara at the root of the lash and unfold the color in a rolling motion.

■ Apply several times while the mascara is wet—don't allow it to dry; don't cake on the color.

■ Not everybody should use mascara on top and bottom lashes. Try just a light brown line beneath the lashes. (That's what I use.)

■ If you do put mascara on your lower lashes, apply with the hand held vertically, and place a facial tissue under the lashes so you don't blotch up your makeup.

■ Black mascara is best for everybody. It

just does the most. Brown is a waste of money, and red, blue and violet are fads.

■ Long-lash types of mascara usually have fibers that can get into your eyes, but they *do* make your lashes appear thicker. I find the best way to apply long-lash mascaras is to first apply a regular one, then use the long-lash. Have a toothbrush or mascara comb nearby in case you need it to separate your lashes before the mascara dries. Remember Maribeth! *Don't* stab yourself.

If your mascara is getting dried out, add a drop of mineral water and mix well. This can save ready-to-be-discarded mascara.

MAKEUP BRUSHES

I'm a big believer in using makeup brushes —it's a more hygienic way to apply makeup and gives a more professional, smooth look. Invest in a set of good brushes, and avoid the applicators that companies provide with their cosmetics. (They're usually made of cheap goods.) Keep your brushes clean: wash with soap and water, soak in Barbicide regularly once a week, then rinse thoroughly. Shape the brush with your fingers while it is wet. If you are having a professional makeup, make sure the brushes used on you have been cleaned properly before they touch your face. Sable brushes are softest and cause the least irritation to sensitive skin (see page 97). Put labels on them so you know which is for what products.

QUICKIE MAKEUP

Everyone should have two makeup plans: the regular everyday, relaxed procedure that takes ten to twenty minutes and a quickie plan that takes no more than five. Some days you just don't have the time for anything more—but with some practice, your quickie routine can be very effective. Anyone can be completely and well made-up in five minutes. I have even done it for two women I had never seen before on the *Merv Griffin Show*. And it will certainly make you look better than if you'd run out of the house with no makeup at all. Here's the routine I follow when I'm pressed for time:

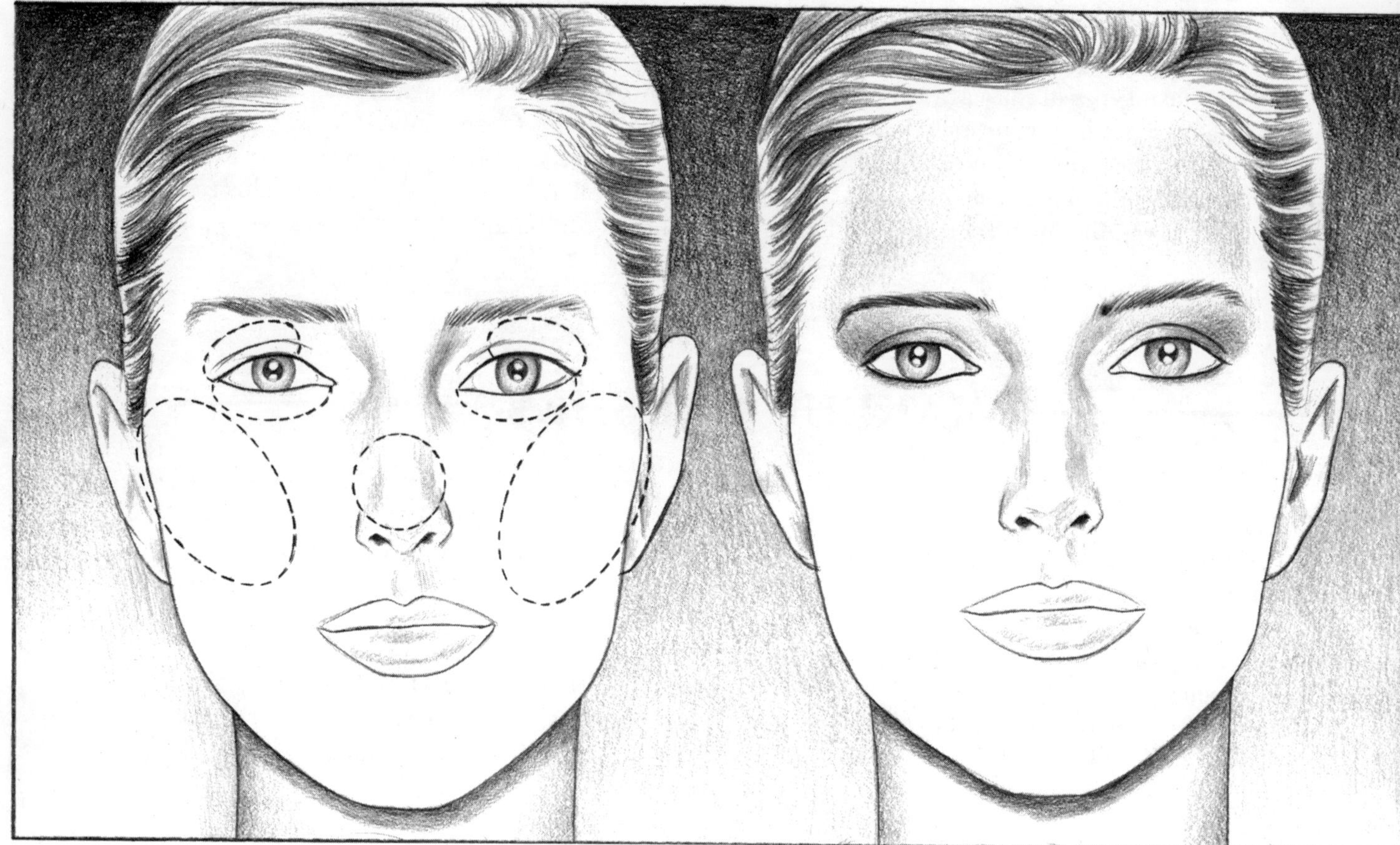

■ Apply moisturizer just where you need it; then under-eye cream.

■ Put foundation only where you need it —if it is exactly matched to your skin, it will blend easily. In my quickie makeup I just put a dab of foundation on my nose and cheeks and blend quickly with a clean sponge. Be sure to put a dab of cream foundation on the eyelids to hold the shadows and under the eyes to conceal dark circles.

■ Apply pale eye shadow from lid up to brows and put a darker color in the crease. I like peach or pink shadow, which others usually use only for highlighting.

■ Outline entire eye with a colored pencil. I like to switch colors and thickness of lines depending on my mood, clothes or the season . . . sometimes I use navy blue or bright blue, dark brown or even summer bright green.

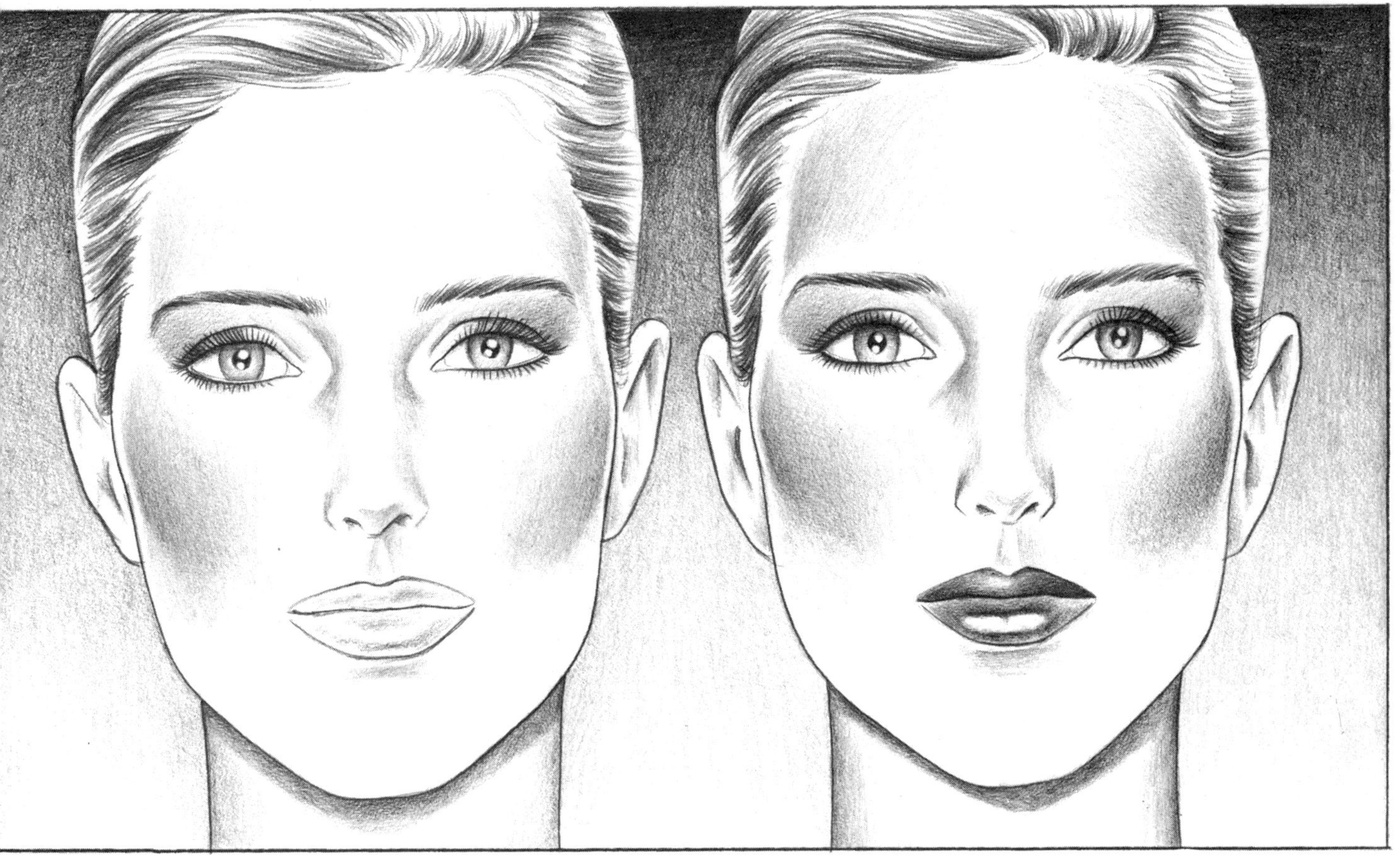

After ringing the eye with color, smudge the color with a Q-tip so it doesn't look severe. Many eye pencils come with their own sponges for smudging. Other people prefer liquid liner because it doesn't smear. You can smudge the liquid before it dries or leave it in a thin line. Experiment before you are in a hurry so you know the best technique for quickie days.

■ Apply mascara. I do just upper lashes.

■ Use a dash of rouge—or skip it if your skin already has a healthy bloom.

■ Finish off with a light brown lip pencil to outline your lips and a clear gloss or a soft color inside it.

CHANGING YOUR SKIN TONE

Lots of people think they can alter their skin color merely by applying a new shade of makeup base. Instead, they end up looking as if they were wearing a mask. Remember, the neck is where you should always match your makeup—no matter what the season or time of day. Then, if you want to add color to your face, use rouge and shadows, but *never* try to change your skin tone through foundation.

If you have freckles you want to cover, select a foundation shade halfway between the color of your neck skin and that of the freckles, and use a sponge to blend smoothly. People who have freckles usually want to hide them; people who don't have freckles think they are cute. This is a lot like the curly-hair/straight-hair syndrome. Frequently people with freckles have fair skin, so be sure not to use an unnaturally dark shade in trying to cover the dots. Foundation is not always necessary—something few seem to realize. You may need it just on the parts of your skin where you are trying to even out the color or to blend in a freckle or discoloration.

To fake a tan with makeup, use a dark liquid foundation with a very light hand and extend the color down the neck. Make sure you don't go too orange or too dark, and blend well. Bronzes are also good. They work best when mixed with a little moisturizer before applying. This reduces streaking and makes application easier. Make sure the product you use is nonstaining and allows the skin underneath to *breathe*.

MAKEUP AS CAMOUFLAGE

Basically, I don't believe in camouflage for pimples or acne. A skin eruption will go away a lot faster if it *isn't* covered, stays clean and can breathe (Makeup traps oils). But if you have a big date, or are making a television appearance, or need to contour your features for a photograph, makeup can certainly create any number of illusions.

If you have circles under your eyes, use a heavier-textured cream foundation to dispel the darkness, or buy a camouflage stick. You should use the shade closest to your own skin color; otherwise it will show through your makeup. Using a color that is too light will not cover dark circles properly and won't blend into your foundation, and you will have a reverse raccoon effect. The under-eye color should be in the same tone as your foundation. Don't use a white cake or cream, even if you have light, light skin. If you have black skin and are prone to darker circles, don't use a pink or orange camouflage.

If your nose is a tad too wide, you can narrow it by shading a slightly darker-color foundation on the sides of the bridge. If it is too long, apply darker color to tip, then apply a lighter shade down the middle. Lighter colors highlight and should be three shades lighter than your foundation. Darker shades recede and should be four shades darker than foundation. Practice shading a lot before you leap into the public eye; if you are too heavy-handed, you'll look like a TV Indian in war paint. Shading is best used for photography rather than real life because it tends to look phony—or dirty—up close.

KATHRYN KLINGER'S BEST MAKEUP TRICKS

■ Anytime you go to a makeup artist, ask her, or him, to write down what she used. That way you can always come back for the products if you decide later that you liked the look. Some artists will even do a chart for you or fill in a partially illustrated face, showing you exactly where to put each color.

■ A few changes in makeup can really give you a psychological boost. Add a couple of new items to your makeup collection once or twice a year whether you need them or not. Spring and fall are good times, or maybe for your birthday. If you are feeling blue, a new lipstick and coordinating blush may make your day bright again.

■ Many women are afraid of bright colors, especially bright lipstick. *Try* one every now and then and see what it does for you—it could be a big improvement.

■ A makeup sponge absorbs pressure, so when you put on makeup you'll get a lighter, sheer look and never clog your pores with a heavy-handed dose of foundation.

■ To "set" an eye-pencil makeup, apply shadow over the pencil with a liner brush.

■ It's fun to mix pencil colors to create your own shade. I often apply a light brown pencil and then go over it with a dark brown pencil. Blue over light brown also looks interesting. I experimented recently with a dark pink lip pencil on my eyes and a bright blue line on top of it. I got a bright purple line. It was great.

■ My favorite eyeliner trick is to line the eye with a very skinny black line (all the way around), then apply color right on top of it. This really brings out the eye and works for top and bottom. If you have watery-looking eyes or thin eyelashes, this is an especially good trick for you.

■ Always coordinate lipstick and rouge to the same color family—rust rouge with peach lipstick is a winner; plum rouge and peach lipstick is a no-no. Peaches, rusts and all oranges belong in the same family; pinks and plums go together; reds can be blended into either group depending on the tone; blue reds belong to the pink family and coral reds to the orange group.

■ Coordinate the depth of color on your face to the amount of color on your body. If your clothes are in hot, vibrant hues, your face needs more of the same, otherwise the clothes will "wear" you. If you are wearing pastels, don't make up a bright face—go soft instead.

■ Combinations of shadows sold in one case are a waste of money. They may be eye-catching in a store, but you will never use all those colors equally; if you run out of the one you use most frequently, you won't want to buy another set just to get that one color. I find it is best to buy single-color containers and replenish as needed. It's also easier to carry one or two small color pots than a big box with shades you never use.

■ A bright lipstick will make your teeth look whiter. If you have less than perfect teeth (or stained teeth), do not wear pale lipstick. The more contrast there is between lips and teeth, the whiter teeth look.

■ Have a white and a beige lipstick on hand so you can create your own shades by combining with the lipsticks you already have.

■ The best way to assess a new eye-makeup look is to do one eye the "old" way and one the "new" way. Which one looks better?

■ Mascara on both upper and lower lashes is not a must. In fact, I find most people look better without mascara on the bottom lashes. Dark lashes cast a shadow under the eyes. Try one eye with and one without to see which looks better on you.

■ If you don't have sensitive eyes, investigate the kind of mascara with nylon fibers in it, which attach to your lashes and make them look longer and fuller. There is another type of fiber that you brush on top of wet mascara. This takes a quick and adept hand so the lashes don't clump together.

■ Pick darker eye-shadow colors; they will always do more for your eyes than pale shades.

■ Today, with Americans becoming more health-conscious and more exercise-oriented, the makeup trend will be toward sheerer bases. Makeup will be used more subtly to make each person look better, not made-up. Use foundation and use blush sparingly—let your natural glow show through. If you have no natural glow, don't try to heighten your complexion with makeup. Go back to Chapters Two and Three and see where you went wrong.

ALLERGY TESTING

Do a patch test to see if you really are allergic to a product before tossing it out. Don't use the product for a couple of days, and clear up the affected area. Then apply the product to a small controlled area, like the middle of your forehead or one of your cheeks. If the problem reappears there, you are certain you're allergic.

Allergies usually burn or itch and often look like uniform little bumps. If you get another kind of breakout from a product, you are not necessarily allergic—it could be another kind of adverse reaction, or that the product is too strong or too oily for your type of skin. Discontinue use, test a week later, then decide. A face cream that makes you break out need not be thrown out—it could be great for your hands or as an after-bath body rub. Return products that cause breakouts to the store or manufacturer. If your allergic reaction was so severe you needed medical help, write the manufacturer and enclose your medical bills. Some companies pay those bills.

WEDDING BELLES

I often see someone new in the salon who will tell me that she's always wanted to come in but was waiting for a special occasion. Now she is getting married and wants to be "made over." While she did come to the right place, she came at the wrong time. Brides should never experiment on *anything* unless they have plenty of time *before* the wedding, not the day before.

For your wedding and the subsequent photographs, you should have a hairdo you know suits you and always looks good; you should wear makeup you feel comfortable in, that makes you look like you. (And the woman he fell in love with.) This is not the time to get a perm, try a new hairstyle, break out some hot new eyeshadow color or wear the latest shade of nail polish you saw in a fashion magazine. You shouldn't even have a facial right before your wedding unless you know exactly how your skin will react.

If your wedding has been planned for months in advance, use that time to do whatever experimenting you want. Try all new colors against white, or the color of your dress or suit. Try hairstyles with the veil or hat you will be wearing. Pick a neutral nail polish color.

Always have a trial run before the wedding. Test your hair and makeup. Use the same hairstylist, the same makeup products and the same makeup artist if you will not be doing your makeup yourself. Take instant pictures of the trial. Study them, experiment. Keep only the pictures that show the perfect version. Use them as cue cards for the big event.

Best hint: Pick floral colors that are "pretty," not fad colors. These shades photograph well and won't date the photos as much as more trendy, extreme palettes may.

MAKEUP PROBLEMS (AND SOLUTIONS)

■ Help! My eye shadow gets smeary and gooey and *never* lasts.

My guess is that you are using pencil shadows—switch to pressed powder and see if you get better results. (I bet you will.) Put foundation on your eyelids so your shadow has a good base. If you work best with pencils, apply powdered shadow over the pencil to set it.

■ Help! What mascara should I wear when I swim?

So-called waterproof mascara is not all it's

cracked up to be. It sometimes clumps lashes together and rarely lasts all day or all dunking. Why wear makeup when you swim? Sunblock should be enough, and don't forget to reapply after the swim.

■ Help! Taking off makeup is just too complicated for me. I tend to be lazy. Any hints?

Use eye makeup remover pads, then face makeup remover, then a toner on your skin. Splash everything off with cold water.

■ Help! How can I stop mascara from messing up my makeup?

Apply mascara only to upper lashes if you have a smearing problem. This will also "open" eyes more. Make sure the wand is not loaded with excess mascara. Comb your lashes gently with an eyebrow comb to get off any extra gobs while mascara is still damp. Do not cake on mascara; this will not help matters and may make lashes break.

■ Help! My eyes are small.

Make your eyes look bigger by using a bright blue eyeliner under the bottom lashes. Some makeup artists will recommend putting the pencil *inside* the eye, but this is iffy and doesn't stay on well. A soft blue line close to the lashes and extended slightly beyond the outer corners will give the illusion of a larger eye. Using darker shadows gives more definition to small eyes. Extend color out and above the lid to the crease to give the impression of larger lid surface. Lots of mascara helps too!

SCARS AND MAKEUP

When I was a junior in college I was in a serious car accident—the tire of the car I was riding in blew out. The car skidded completely across six lanes of highway and ended up in a ditch. I was wearing a seat belt and, luckily, no one in the car was seriously injured. An ambulance took us to the local county hospital and there, in the emergency room, I found myself covered with blood from gashes under my chin and across my forehead.

I was stitched up right away, too stunned even to think of asking for a plastic surgeon. The doctor who sewed me up did an adequate job and, over the years, the scar has improved. I suspect that I, alone, am aware of it—especially when I have makeup on.

The first facial scars a person receives are traumatic. If you have such an injury, here are a few tips for beautiful healing and hiding:

■ If you are not in a life-and-death situation, ask for a plastic surgeon rather than the regular emergency doctor.

■ While the stitches are in, don't try to cover the wound with makeup or hair or anything else. Wounds need to be kept clean and to heal.

■ When the stitches are taken out, ask your doctor when you can apply makeup. Usually the skin is still raw and needs additional healing time.

■ Don't touch a healing wound. Your chances of scarring are greater if you touch and inadvertently remove a scab. You can also get an infection.

■ When you are ready to camouflage a scar, use a heavy-textured cream foundation on the scar area only. Blend it well with a clean sponge, then apply your own foundation over it. Use a pressing motion and don't rub.

Remember:

■ The finesse of the doctor shows in your healing. Especially if you have elective surgery, choose a good plastic surgeon—even for removing moles or warts from your face. Raised scars are harder to cover than flat ones—the work of a good doctor can make a big difference!

■ Don't be a heroine. If you need stitches, get them.

Scars can occur, even with the best medical care, from simple dermatological procedures like removing a growth. They can be white or red. If you have a small growth that isn't cancerous and isn't dangerous, leave well enough alone.

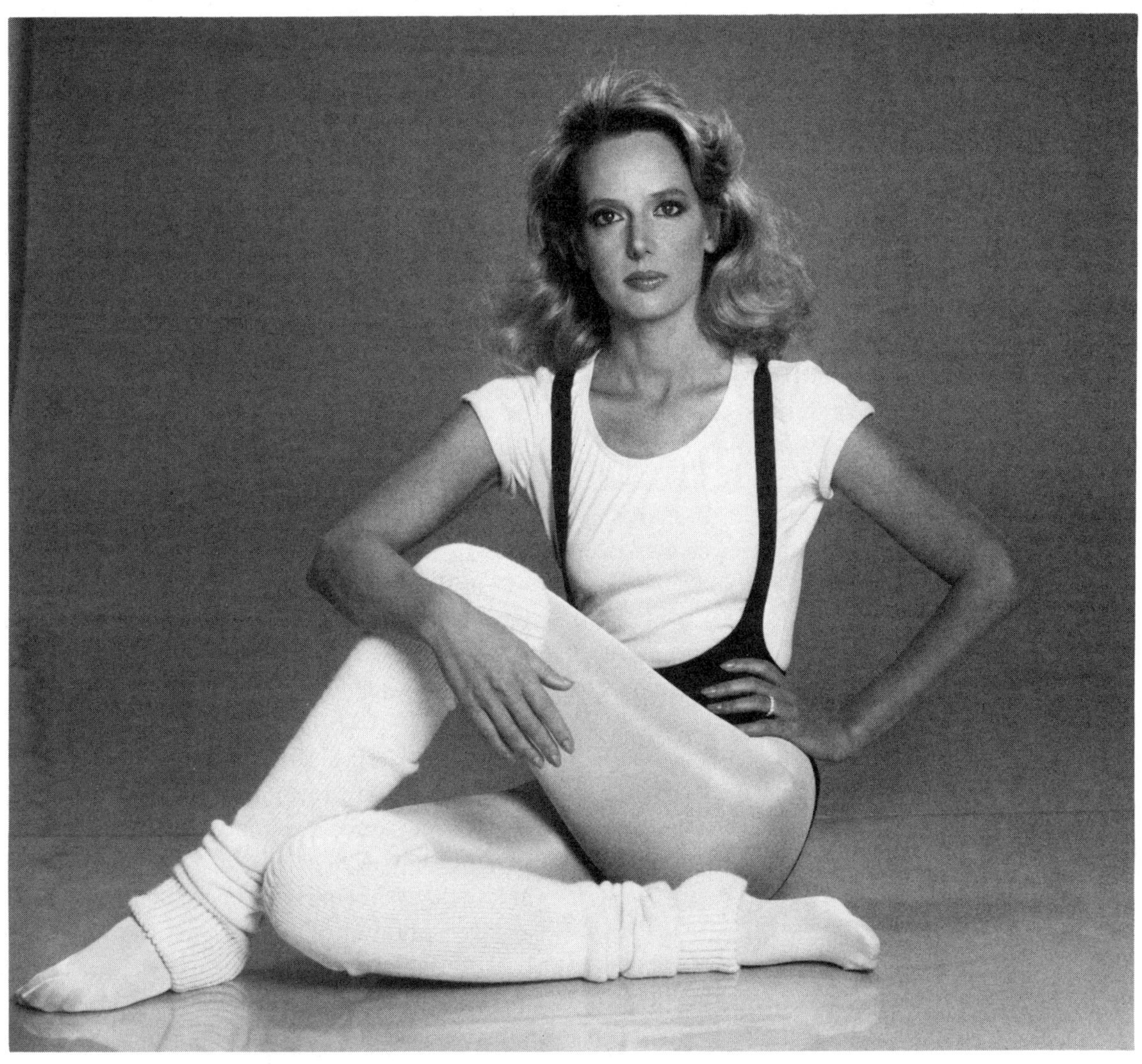

Nine

Plastic Surgery

BEYOND CAMOUFLAGE

If you really have a structural flaw in your face that makeup cannot fix (and believe me, makeup *can* do wonders), you may be ready to consider plastic surgery.

Plastic surgery is a very personal thing. Some people spend years fantasizing about it. Others think it's bad luck to play around with what God gave them. Surgery has been known to make people happy and change their lives for the better; it can leave others confused, bewildered or dissatisfied.

Generally speaking, my own philosophy is to leave well enough alone, *unless* you are totally preoccupied with a specific cosmetic problem. Cosmetic surgery is not a perfect science. You always take a risk—scars, complications, mistakes. *But* if all you can think about is your big nose or your Dumbo ears and you have reached obsession point, then you are probably a good candidate for surgery.

My friend Lillian, the one so perfect she made angels nervous, had her nose fixed after high school. "I'm so happy I got rid of my W. C. Fields nose," she told me with pride. I promise you there was nothing wrong with Lillian's nose before her surgery, and the change was barely perceptible to anyone except Lillian and her mother. Yet it turned out that all her young life Lillian had been obsessed with her nose, and whether she actually needed surgery or not, she *thought* she did.

In Lillian's case, the surgery was successful, and she has never again complained about a single feature in her perfect face or body. However, there are some people who use plastic surgery as a substitute for solving their life's problems. They think "everything will be all right" once they have transformed that offending part of their anatomy. The surgery once completed, they then think either that the doctor did a crummy job or that yet *another* part of their body needs fixing or replacing. They are never happy and go from one doctor to another, seeking a satisfaction they will never find because the help they need is psychological, not surgical.

OFFICE VS. HOSPITAL PLANS

As medicine becomes more and more advanced, many doctors are able to perform delicate surgical procedures in their offices. Patients often prefer this because it:

■ cuts expenses drastically;

■ is not as traumatic as checking into a hospital.

While I am no lover of hospitals, I do recommend that if you are having cosmetic surgery, you have it done in one. In the rare case where there are complications, all the emergency equipment the doctor needs is right at his fingertips.

If you are indeed interested in saving money, ask if you can have the surgery done in a hospital on an outpatient basis. You will not be spending the night there, so you will save. Or perhaps you can go home shortly after the surgery and have spent only a single night in the hospital. The shorter the stay, the less expensive.

CHOOSING DR. RIGHT

The best way to find a plastic surgeon is by word of mouth and actual look-see meetings with former patients. If someone you know mentions having surgery, ask about the doctor and the procedure.

Plastic surgeons usually practice in the larger cities, so if you live in a small town, you might well want to investigate several doctors in the nearest metropolis. In the United States, New York and Beverly Hills are the plastic-surgery capitals, but there are excellent surgeons in other cities.

If you don't know anyone to recommend a doctor to you, ask your internist to make suggestions; check with the most reputable hospitals in the city where you want to have the surgery performed. It's best to get a doctor who has made a good reputation for himself but is not yet world-famous. Doctors who get a lot of publicity or who ride on old reputations may not always do the best job for you.

I am very picky about this, but I like plastic surgeons who shy away from publicity, who do not have reputations as playboys (some do) and who voluntarily announce that they don't drink. A doctor's doctor is always a good choice. I think it makes a big difference in the doctor's patience and mood if he doesn't drink. And you know his hands will be steady.

After you've narrowed your list of prospective surgeons down to about three, go visit them in person and have a consultation. (Some charge for this, others don't—ask when you make the appointment.) Ask to see Before and After pictures of former patients. Doctors may be reluctant to tell you the names of their patients, but they will show you pictures and will often show you their charitable work.

Ask the doctor what he suggests for you; he or she may even give you a sketch. Look around the reception area and talk to other patients; ask the receptionist if you can talk to some former patients or get a good look at their faces. Often the doctor has performed surgery on someone in his office and you can get a good close look. My friend Lorraine was so careful she was determined to see at least one nose job done by her potential doctor. The receptionist was kind enough to invite her to her house to see her two daughters, who had been recent patients.

Get *at least three opinions* before you choose the doctor, and compare prices as well as methods. Very few will turn away prospective clients, so it's your job to do as much research as you can. If you find a doctor who actually says you don't need the surgery you are considering, respect his opinion. This is an honest physician who is not money-hungry. You're probably better off without the procedure.

When you interview, be sure to ask who will actually be doing the work. You don't want to be surprised in the operating room to find another doctor or an assistant doing the surgery. Believe me, this happens! I've seen two doctors who work together and the sides of the patient's face don't match! Tell your doctor that you want only him or her to operate on you. Speak up . . . before it's too late.

TO TELL THE TRUTH

Some people are very proud of their plastic surgery and like to tell everyone about it. Others will deny they have had it, no matter how hard you press. Telling is up to you—after all, this is an intensely personal matter and some people are more private than others.

If you decide *not* to tell, make sure you can get away with it. If Barbra Streisand had her signature nose turned overnight into a Bob Hope ski-jump, she would have a hard time denying she had had any surgery. If, however, she had several small operations over a period of years and never said a word, she could probably reshape her nose substantially and get away with it.

The trick to going undiscovered is to make a small change and to go out of town immediately afterward. Then choose a new hairstyle or hair color, so if anyone says you look a little different, quickly point out that you've changed your coiffure.

PLASTICS, BENJAMIN

Plastic surgery is more than skin-deep. It is always a risk. Do not take such a big step lightly. You must have parental consent if you are under twenty-one. Investigate the doctors and procedures thoroughly. Be an *informed* patient. In fact, there are some psychotherapists whose specialty is dealing with patients who have had—or are contemplating—plastic changes. I talked to Dr. Karen L. Fritts in Los Angeles, who gave me this list of tips for the prospective patient:

Before surgery

1. *Examine your expectations.* Self-examination should begin way before the interviewing process. Ask yourself what is your wish. A lot of people don't make conscious what they are expecting, or even why they are about to walk into an operating room. Are your expectations realistic? Do you think the surgery will significantly change your life? Do you fully understand that the surgeon cannot alter your insides and your feelings, that it is only the shape of a nose or a breast that will be changed?

2. *Ask "for whom" questions of yourself.* For whom are you actually having this done? A lot of fourteen- and fifteen-year-olds end up having plastic surgery because their parents want it for them. Inside, the teenagers are more confused by the feelings of rejection and inadequacy ("I'm not pretty enough for Mom") than having any feelings of deformity or unhappiness with an imperfect feature. In the next age bracket, a lot of surgery is done to attract men. Later on, women may consider plastic surgery to keep their husbands from looking at younger girls or to prevent a man from leaving them —both bad reasons. If surgery is "other-oriented," rethink it.

3. *Say goodbye.* People need to say goodbye to the changing parts of their bodies. You don't just throw away a part casually, or give yourself into the hands of a surgeon and order up a new you without taking the time to adjust psychologically. Say goodbye to the old part in order to say hello to the new. It is very troublesome to go into surgery without realizing that you are *losing* as well as adding. Post-surgical depression may be avoided with proper mourning *before* surgery.

After surgery

It takes time to get to know the new you. Integrate your new appearance with your personality. Meet your new feature and plug it into your sense of self. It can be very confusing when you look into a mirror and see change. Successful surgical patients have, within two to three years, integrated the changes to the point that they feel they have *always* looked this way, *always* felt this way about themselves.

NOSES

A "nose job" is technically called rhinoplasty. Most people have their noses "fixed" for cosmetic reasons, although there are several medical reasons to have this surgery done—like obstructed breathing.

The nose does not reach its full size until age fifteen or sixteen, so a nose job should not be considered before that time. The surgeon studies pictures of the patient's face, takes measurements and decides how to rebuild the nose. All the incisions are done inside, so there are no outside scars. The nose can be de-bumped or made shorter, longer, wider or narrower. Sometimes the cartilage needs to be broken in two different places so the doctor can work his magic. This is a slightly more difficult and time-consuming procedure.

The rebuilt nose is usually put in a splint for twenty-four to forty-eight hours, then taped in place for a few days. The area around the eyes is usually black-and-blue for a few weeks. You may not be able to wear glasses or contact lenses for a week or two. Noses usually take a full year to fully "settle" and for swelling to totally disappear.

Nose surgery is the most common type of plastic surgery, and when performed for cosmetic reasons it is done more frequently on young women than on young men. Dona had a nose just like her mother's. While this large hooked beak had never bothered her mother, Dona was obsessed with changing hers. Her family could not afford a fancy plastic surgeon, and the only way she could have it done was through the V.A. hospital where her father was on staff.

"You could come out looking worse than when you go in," Dona's mother warned her. In fact, so upset was she about the surgery that when she took Dona to the hospital and signed the consent form, she fainted. Convinced she could never come out worse, Dona went ahead with the surgery, knowing full well that the job would probably not be done as perfectly as she would like. "I figured *any* improvement would be a help, and that later on, if I needed a second nose job, I could have refinements done when I was out of college and making money." For her sixteenth birthday she had the surgery and received a much smaller, though hardly sophisticated, nose. (It looked like the standard nose job and was very rounded at the tip and the nostrils.) But Dona was thrilled and felt that at least now she had a fighting chance of competing in her peer group. Maybe she would never be the prettiest girl in the class, but she wouldn't have to feel like the class freak either. A few years after she had her original surgery, she was able to go to a well-known specialist in New York and have her nose rebuilt. And now she *is* the prettiest girl on the block.

Shanna had the opposite problem. She had her nose fixed by an expert in Beverly Hills when she was eighteen (She and her mother flew in from Kansas City because of this particular doctor's excellent reputation), and she *loved* her new nose and the look it gave her. She became a professional model and was known as a great beauty in fashion and retailing circles. When she was about thirty-five, without telling anyone, Shanna went to another plastic surgeon and had her cute, *retroussé* nose redone. "As I got older, I felt uncomfortable looking like a teenager. I had developed my own character and my own style, and I wanted a nose that helped my face look like a real face. A perfect little nose seemed like a joke. I certainly didn't want my old nose back, but I wanted something with more character. I feel more sophisticated now that I have had more work done. It's sort of like getting a divorce—that teenage nose was a very good nose for many years, but I've grown into something else." Remember the nose creates balance in the face, and is very important to an individual's character.

Nose-Job Parameters

Age: any age after 16
most commonly performed between ages 16 and 30
Cost: \$3,000 to \$5,000
Where: hospital or office
Length of operation: 2–4 hours.

CHIN IMPLANTS

Often when you have your nose fixed, you'll find that the doctor will recommend a chin implant as well. Or you just may have a facial structure so angular that you appear to have no chin at all, and an implant would help round out the shape of your face. However, if your chin never bothered you and an implant is suggested, your doctor could be trying to get a higher fee.

An implant involves the placement of a high-grade surgical-plastic form that will define the jawline and bring the chin forward. After the surgery a tight bandage is applied for about ten days and a soft-food diet is required. There is a good bit of discomfort for the first day or two, and some discoloration of the skin for a few weeks. The incision is made inside the mouth, so there is no scar. There is rarely infection, complications are minimal and this surgery is considered very low-risk.

"All my life I felt worthless," admits Kara, now in her early thirties. "My mother was beautiful and I was ugly. It was that simple. I got through life by making great grades and being the family scholar. My self-esteem was terribly low, but I never thought much about it. Then, after I was divorced, I decided to pull myself together. I went for makeup and beauty consultations to several experts and plastic surgeons. I had the chin implant done, and a little work on my nose, too, because the doctor said it would balance my face better, and I can't tell you the difference it has made in my life. I know I didn't do it sooner because I just wasn't ready. But I am a changed person now, and I'm loving every minute of it.''

Chin-Implant Parameters

Age: with nose job or any age over 16
Cost: $1,500–$3,000
Where: hospital or office
Length of operation: 1–2 hours

EAR SURGERY

Ear surgery is more often considered for men, but is not uncommon for young women and even for children. No one likes to get teased about having Dumbo ears!

Having your ears ''pinned'' is called otoplasty. It's a simple operation that can be performed on just about anyone over the age of five (the ear has done most of its growing by that time). An incision is made behind the ear; cartilage is reshaped; you are stitched back up and are out of the hospital in a day or two. The stitches are removed in about two weeks, and the patient wears a ski-type mask to sleep in for about six weeks.

There was a girl named Victoria who transferred into my school class from Germany, where her father was stationed in the Army. Victoria was tall and had thick, straight blond hair which she wore in bangs and a one-length cut that was kept behind her ears. She had pierced ears, wore trendy earrings and was Miss Popularity. Everyone in school wanted a ''Vicky Cut,'' but no one's hair was thick enough or straight enough, so no one could quite look like her—though a lot tried. Then, at a slumber party, Victoria confided to me that she wore her famous hairstyle to show off her cute ears. She showed me how small and flat and tight against her head they were—and guess what: at the Army hospital in Germany, she had had her ears operated on! She had always felt ugly when her ears stuck out farther than her braids and had prevailed upon her parents to let her have plastic surgery.

The Ear-Pin Parameters

Age: any age over 5
Cost: $1,000–$2,500
Where: office or hospital
Length of operation: 1–2 hours

DERMABRASION

Dermabrasion is a type of surgery that removes the top layer of skin to help clear up acne scars or to make you look younger without having a face lift. Essentially the skin is frozen, then sanded off. It emerges red and raw and has to heal. It heals with new skin, and the hope is that the new skin will look better than the old. But meanwhile there are many drawbacks: The process is expensive, painful and inconvenient—before the new skin grows back, your face is raw and scabbed. You cannot ever again go out in the sun; your skin will be very prone to discoloring. And you have no idea what the new skin will look like; you may come out looking like a princess—or a frog. It's a high-risk procedure. It's possible for the actual color of your skin to change, and your face and neck may not match in color. Also, the acne pits may never disappear. I don't recommend this process unless you are desperate.

Linda had terrible acne and spent most of her adolescence hiding from her peers. When she was nineteen she persuaded her parents to let her have dermabrasion. She was lucky and now has perfect skin. Few of her friends know how she suffered during her youth.

Dermabrasion Parameters

Age: teens and up
Cost: $1,200–$3,000
Where: doctor's office
Length of operation: 45 minutes–2 hours

BETTER BREASTS

Size and shape of breasts are psychological matters as well as physical ones because of society's emphasis on breast beauty. And no one seems to be happy with what she has!

Alexandra was a petite woman with overlarge breasts who felt very self-conscious about her chest. She told me she always thought that when people were looking at her face they were making an effort *not* to stare at her chest. She longed for breast-reduction surgery, but all her friends told her she was crazy and to enjoy her full figure. Even her boyfriend (who was insecure and liked having her dependent on him) advised against surgery. Then one day I saw Alexandra in the salon and she asked me if I noticed anything new. I didn't. "I'm wearing a red silk blouse," she announced. When I didn't get her point, she whispered, "I had the surgery, and I've gone from a size fourteen blouse to an eight and I can wear bright colors without being embarrassed." Alexandra's life was made better by an operation even her closest friends had discouraged. "It's such a relief to feel like a normal person," she said.

Yet women who think their breasts are too small have a hard time relating to Alexandra's problem. Luckily, you can have surgery to reduce *or* enlarge breasts, depending on your needs. (You can also have what's called breast reconstruction if you've had a mastectomy.)

Creating larger breasts is called breast augmentation, and each year about 200,000 women in this country have it done. The operation has become sophisticated and is far safer than when first invented. (Some women had *sponges* implanted in their breasts in the early 1960s!) A breastlike form, usually an envelope filled with salt water or silicone, is inserted into the breast over the chest muscles.

The most important factor in choosing a larger breast is getting a believable size. A lot depends on how much skin is available. A thin, flat-chested woman cannot turn into Bo Derek even with the help of a gifted surgeon.

Breast reduction is performed on women whose breasts have stretched out of shape after pregnancy and nursing or on women who were just plain overendowed. Too heavy a set of breasts can cause backache and poor posture—as well as psychological damage. To make breasts smaller, the surgeon makes an incision around the areola of the nipple; skin, subcutaneous fat and breast tissue are removed. There is some scarring, but on most people it heals over a period of time. Again, I know I'm square, but I must say leave well enough alone whenever possible. A lot of horror stories are true stories.

Breast-Reduction Parameters

Age: 21 or over
Cost: $3,000–$5,000
Where: office or hospital
Length of operation: 2–4 hours

Breast-Augmentation Parameters

Age: 21 or over
Cost: $3,000–$5,000
Where: office or hospital
Length of operation: 2–4 hours

OTHER OPERATIONS

There are many other types of plastic surgery. Some are performed primarily for cosmetic reasons, like having drooping eyelids resculpted, or creating tighter skin via a face lift. There is also reconstructive plastic surgery for people with burns or hereditary deformities. Accident victims often need many sessions in the operating room with a skilled surgeon.

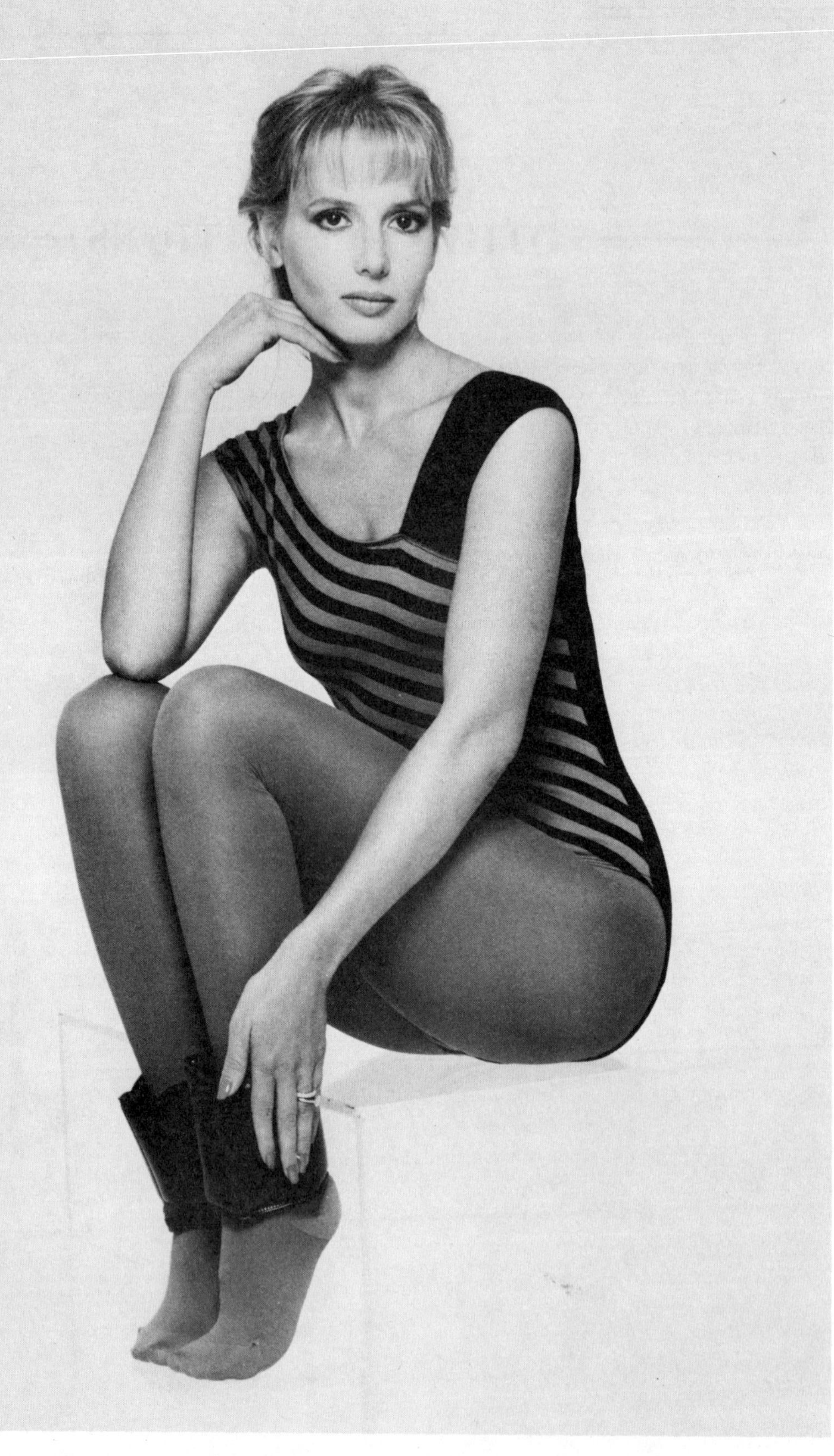

Ten

Health and Exercise

BODY TALK

The type of body you have is probably inherited. I inherited one of the more carefree ones, the mesomorphic. However, I spent many years disguising my ideal shape because I got *lazy.* Not only did I get thunder thighs and a flabby seat, but I went through a phase of looking like a stuffed sausage!

There are three basic body types:

- *Ectomorph*—the tall, thin person with long limbs and muscles who has trouble gaining weight;
- *Mesomorph*—the muscular, athletic type with broad shoulders tapering to a narrow waist;
- *Endomorph*—the shorter, pear-shaped, more rounded person who must always watch weight.

This is not to say that there aren't any svelte endomorphs, or that mesomorphs have it made in the shade. Anyone can blow it! (I did!) And that's when I discovered the worst news: it's *harder* to get back into shape than it is to keep it. No matter what your body type, you'll find *staying* in shape is the best alternative—mentally and physically. Endomorphs may have trouble reducing their curves, and ectomorphs have to work hard to gain muscle definition, but once you get in shape and stay in shape, it's worth it!

My basic philosophy of weight control is to *stay the same weight throughout your life.* I don't mean that if you're 287 pounds you should stay there! Find a realistic weight suitable to your body type. If you have had a weight problem since childhood, use your later teen years to get it under control; then spend the rest of your life dedicated to keeping your weight stable. If you're already past your teen years, there's no better time to get to work on yourself than now! It will be harder to get your figure under control as each day passes, so stop wasting time and start using some discipline. Take it off and keep it off. The "yo-yo" syndrome of repeated weight gain and loss is bad for all body types (although it plagues endomorphs most) and should be avoided by conscientious weight control practiced every day of your life. How?

Discipline.

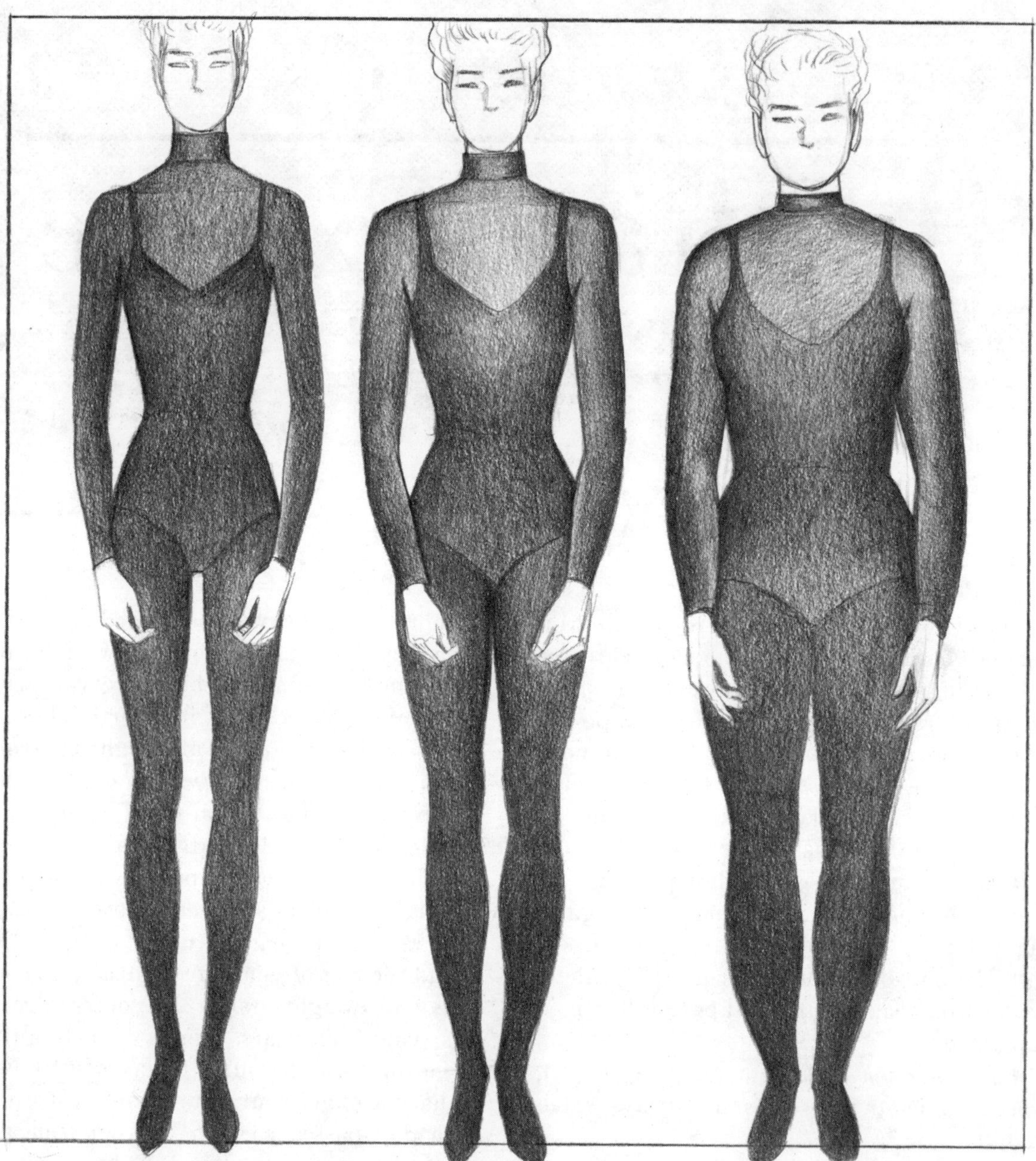

Ectomorph *Mesomorph* *Endomorph*

First thing each day: weigh yourself when you get up. If you are a pound over, lose it! If you get three pounds over, go out and buy a three-pound steak and take a good look at all that bulk. Visualize those three mean pounds. Realize that three pounds can make a difference in how your clothes fit. Three can become five very easily, and then you'll have a bigger problem. Take the weight off immediately. Nothing is worse for your body or your skin tone than adding and shedding weight your whole life long.

I have a personal slogan to remind me of the struggle to stay thin: Inside every skinny person is a fat person trying desperately *not* to get out!

People envy the thin person, but most thin people have to work at staying that way, whether they admit to it or not. The older we get, the harder it is to stay thin and the more discipline figure control requires. A young metabolism can get away with a few sins (junk food, dessert, you know), but between ages twenty-five and thirty, the body changes—then it takes work and discipline to keep a good figure if you haven't neglected your figure in the first place. If you've been careless with your shape and want to get back to basics, it takes *lots* of work and *lots* of discipline.

EAT RIGHT

The key to eating right is to eat food from the four food groups—fruit/vegetable; bread/cereal; meat/poultry/fish; dairy—and never to eat a portion larger than a clenched fist.

Drink lots of water (probably bottled unless you know your tap water is healthful) and avoid fast foods, junk foods, greasy and fatty foods and too much red meat.

My daily food plan looks something like this:

Breakfast

(I believe in a large breakfast; it'll reduce your chances of getting a headache later in the day.)

winter: 1 egg with bacon
fresh fruit
an 8-oz. glass of the fresh-squeezed juice of 4 oranges
an 8-oz. glass of water
no coffee or tea

Note: It's better to drink the water 15–30 minutes before breakfast to clean out the system.

summer: bran cereal with raisins and low-fat milk
½ sliced banana
an 8-oz. glass of the fresh-squeezed juice of 2 grapefruits
an 8-oz. glass of water
no coffee or tea

Lunch

I take plain sliced fresh veggies to work in a Baggie (no dressing! no salt!).

If I'm having a business lunch, I eat fish or a salad and no dessert or coffee or tea. I drink only bottled water.

Dinner

If I had a business lunch, a light dinner; otherwise, I eat anything I want for dinner, as long as it's healthful; more bottled water (at least 8 oz., maybe 16 oz.).

■ I drink wine with dinner only with guests and rarely have a more alcoholic drink.

■ If I've been really good about all this I think I deserve a dessert, so I indulge! (It's usually chocolate.)

■ Once a week I have a totally vegetarian day. I tell my husband in advance so he can plan a hearty lunch.

CUTTING BACK

I have two techniques for cutting down on the *amount* of food I eat. If I am a few pounds overweight:

■ I eat carefully calculated portions—*never larger than a clenched fist,* smaller if I'm cutting back.

■ I never finish everything on the plate.

When I go out, I often order something I'm not crazy about so I don't mind leaving most of it. Even at home, I'll have something my husband likes that I don't care for, so I won't be tempted to eat too much. It's much harder to leave your favorite food on the plate.

How a food is prepared has a lot to do with how fattening it is, so go simple and reap the rewards. Broiled or grilled is always better than fried; raw veggies are better than cooked; steamed are better than boiled. Most people are not honest about what they eat. Some are actually lying to themselves; others just make "little" social fibs. Or they talk a lot about their "metabolism" and how it affects their figures. But gaining weight is rarely the result of a metabolism problem—you gain weight when you eat more than you burn off. Each person is different, so too much is a matter of what is too much for *you.*

POSTURE

I have a client who is an extremely successful woman—she dresses in expensive designer clothes, carries a $300 handbag and wears diamond stud earrings day and night. She has a pretty face, makes herself up well and should be everyone's idea of Superwoman. But because she has bad posture, because of her rounded shoulders and stooped-over carriage, she looks like a loser instead of the winner she really is.

Good posture should be developed from childhood. It is far harder to correct posture once it has eroded, but it can be done. Posture is largely a function of the lower back muscles, the abdominal muscles and the shoulders, so these muscle groups must be worked on, strengthened and developed to hold the body upright. Good posture also helps your body function better, makes you look thinner and feel more poised.

Proper posture means your head is up; chin is up and parallel to feet; back is upright and straight; shoulders back and down; tummy is tucked in; seat is tucked

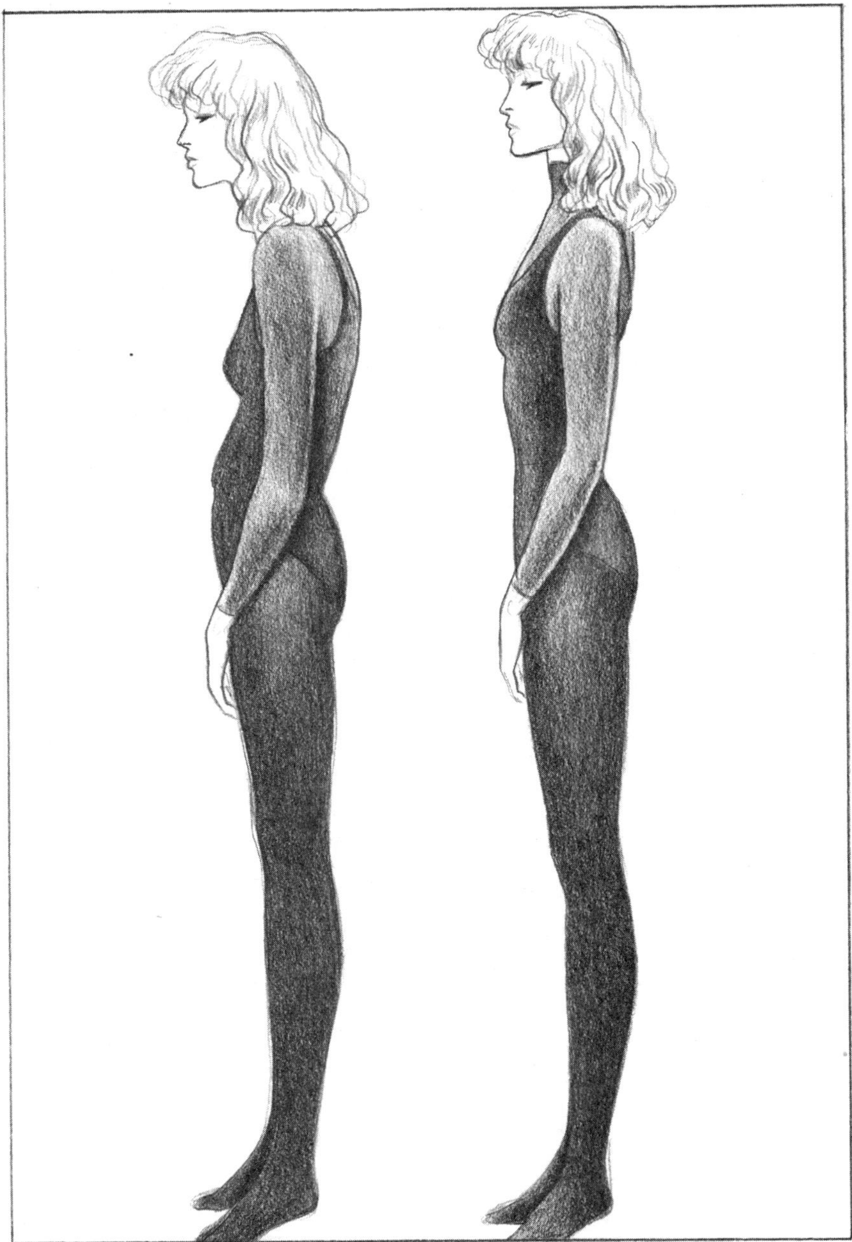

under. In and under, up and back. If your shoulders hunch forward, the spinal cord begins to shorten and the muscles surrounding it become weak—your stomach may even become flabby and you can develop swayback. Thighs and seat spread because the muscles that should keep them tucked in aren't being worked properly. Not carrying your head up can create a double chin and creased neck. If you slouch, you also tend to look down at your feet rather than ahead when you are walking. You can miss an awful lot of the world this way!

Tension often causes bad posture, so if you feel yourself tightening in the neck and shoulders, or hunching over your desk to alleviate back pain, take a break and do some exercises or go for a walk to shake out your muscles. Always sit with your back supported, and move forward from your hips rather than by rounding your spine.

Try this posture helper: Get a long broom, remove the broom, use the stick. By placing the stick behind your shoulders and reaching up to hold it horizontal you will automatically have your shoulders in good posture. Your neck will be straight and in position. Tuck in your tummy and seat, and practice walking. About 3–5 minutes two times a day should help tremendously.

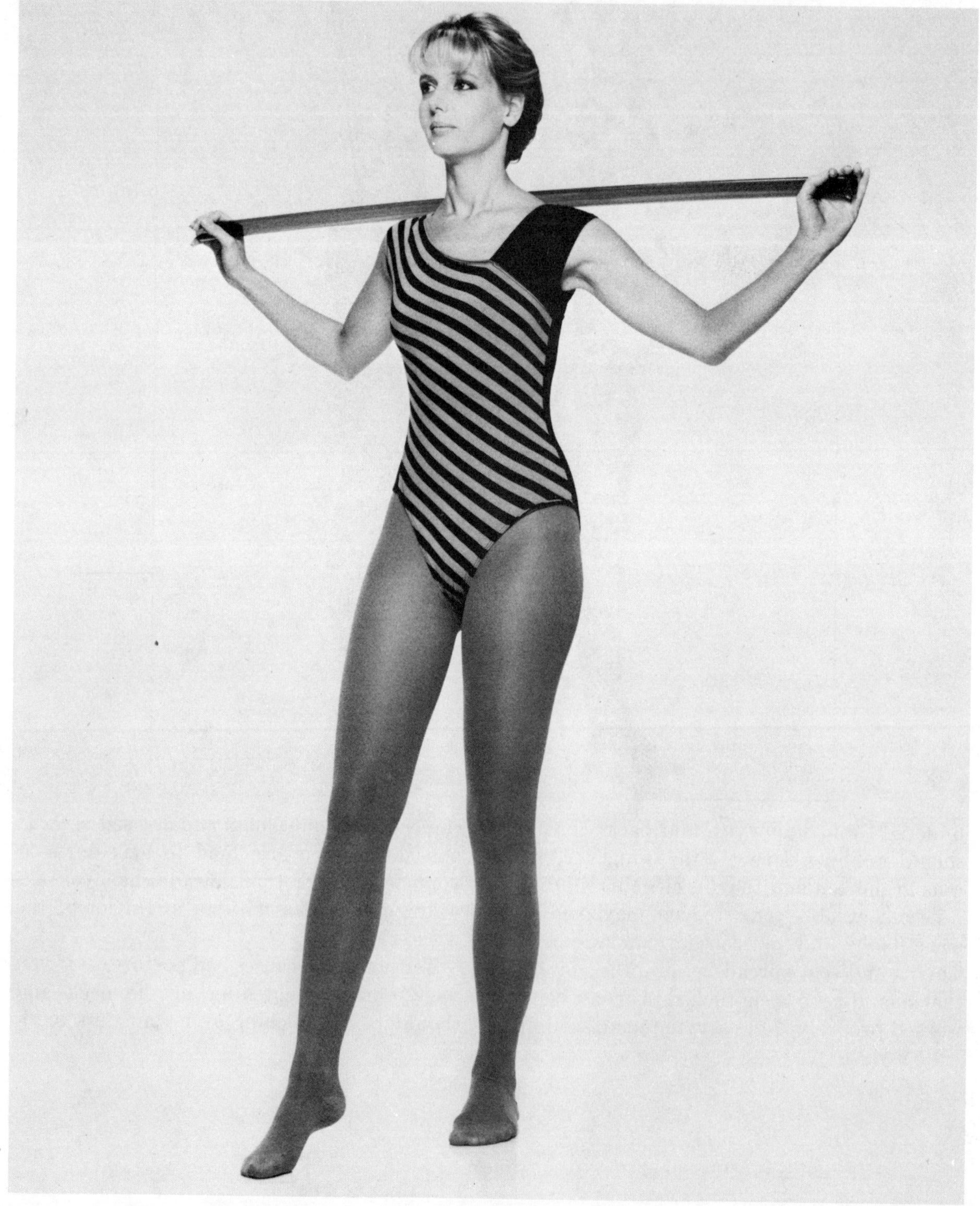

Now try my headlifts: This exercise is a neck strengthener and an important anti-aging exercise. Ten repetitions are plenty. Lie face down, hands one over the other cushioning your head (beneath the forehead is best). Lift your head up off your hands *without* changing your chin position. Then lower forehead back to your hands.

Variation: when forehead is raised, look right, then center (which means look down at the floor); then left, then center.

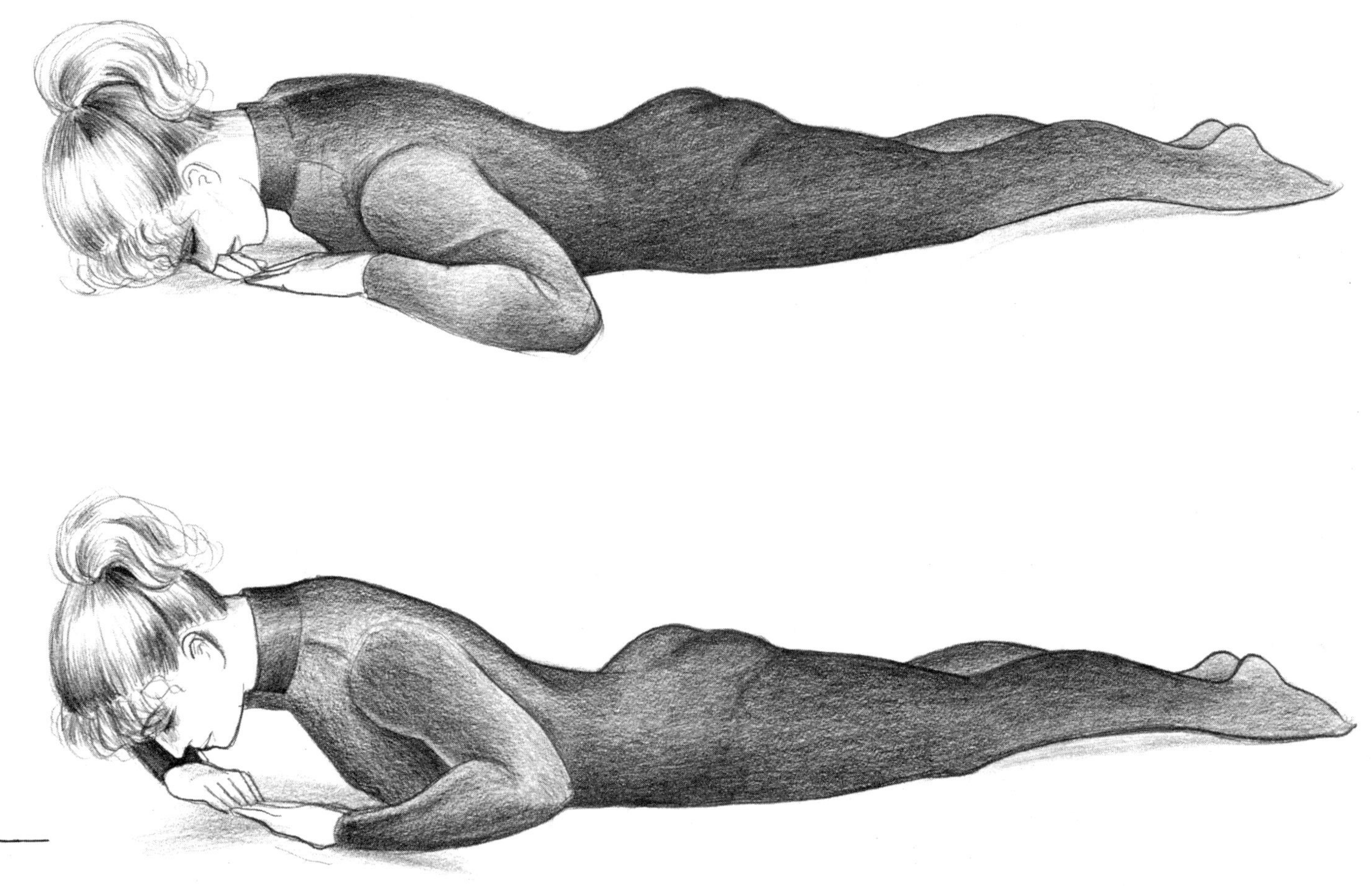

EXERCISING: MY PERSONAL WORK-OFF

It's not that I like to exercise.

I don't.

Once I'm actually doing it, I don't mind, and afterward I love the fact that I've *done* it. But if I can come up with an excuse to worm out of class, I will. In fact, I became so delinquent that I had to come up with my own home program or the exercise truant officer would have come after me.

And still it's hard. There are many mornings I'd rather not.

If I didn't take my weights out and set up my mat between my bed and the bathroom so that I would inevitably trip on them in getting from one important place to the other, I would still have flabby thighs and a rear end suitable only for a sofa.

Even though I exercise just about every day of my life (I even have a special Sunday routine), it is not a habit I slip into like a second skin. I would much rather be eating Edelweiss's chocolate-covered marshmallows and reading a good book.

I grew up in Manhattan, where the only athletic thing a person ever did was walk a few blocks. (This was *before* jogging.) I didn't even learn to ride a bike until I went to college! I played an occasional game of tennis, but even this came to an abrupt halt in my early twenties when I developed a serious knee problem (either from tennis or from eight-inch platform shoes—we never knew which, so I had to give up both!) that put me in extreme pain and sent me on a parade from one specialist to another. I had injections, I had electric-current treatments, I had physical therapy. Nothing helped a problem that was so severe I actually cried every time I had to sit down. Then I went to Dr. James Nicholas, who was the Jets' team doctor, and he saved me. He gave me a series of exercises to do twice a day, with weights. I did them religiously (even shlepping those heavy 15-pound weights on trips and never warning the bellman why my luggage was so heavy) and cured my problem. The basic principle was to develop the rest of my leg and take the pressure off my knee—of course, you had to treat both legs, not just the afflicted one, or the legs would have ended up being two different sizes.

For four years I did my double exercises and was then considered cured. There was just one hitch: I had developed *huge* thighs.

But I wasn't complaining because, after all, I was cured. So for the next ten years, I did nothing.

Nothing isn't completely accurate.

I signed up for a lot of exercise classes with various girlfriends, who would go to a few classes, then quit. If the girlfriend wouldn't go, I wouldn't go. I'm just not motivated to go by myself—I get lonely; I like company. I worked through everyone I knew, on both coasts. And while I was busy joining and dodging, my derriere was getting wider and my once-strong thighs were turning to flab.

Even my own mother, who never criticized me, suddenly began to nag. She said my "seat" was getting big and I had better do something about it.

I tried jogging. It was boring. I tried swimming. I hated getting wet. I tried tennis. I never had time to get a court. I signed up for more exercise classes. No one would go with me. Or I couldn't find a parking spot.

All this time, my seat was not getting any smaller.

So I decided to develop my own plan, designed to meet my needs and to work off the flab that was accumulating at an ominously fast pace. I call it my Work-Off (because it works off those unpleasant ripples), and I like it because:

- I can do it at home—there's no driving time lost; there's no clothes-changing time lost; there's no fighting for a court or dealing with an overcrowded class;
- I'm in control of the amount of time. I can do a lot or a little;
- I can actually control the part of my body that I want to work on next by the way I set up the Work-Off;
- I can wear whatever I want (usually nothing; leotards and tights are flattering);
- I'm not lonely because I'm not uncomfortable—I'm in familiar surroundings, secure in where I am as opposed to feeling alone in a class of strangers who can all do the exercises better;
- I compete only against myself, so I don't have to keep up with the class or worry that everyone else is laughing at me;
- It requires just a little room. I do not have a room in my house built into a gym;
- It's always clean! I can't tell you how many exercise clubs I've been to that had a sweaty, none-too-sanitary feel to them. At some places the carpets are so grimy you can't even *imagine* lying down on them!
- I can do it on the road in my hotel room without having to find a health club. (My job demands a good amount of travel);
- It's FREE!
- There's one other great side effect that I never thought of—I have a stronger body! Knowing that I now have strong legs, I can attempt sports I never considered before. I'm proud I've come this far. I have the body confidence I never had before.

GETTING READY

Every time I signed up for a new exercise class, in all those years when I went sporadically to class, I would always buy myself a new leotard to help motivate me. There's a national craze for rushing out and buying new active wear and sports equipment, often when you don't need it or aren't going to use it. Here are some tips that may save you some money, and the embarrassment of having a closet filled with clothes and equipment you never use:

- Make sure you have an exercise mat. Buy one if need be.
- Exercise naked. (I do.) Then you can be reminded of exactly why you are going through all this torture. There's no real *need* to spend money on leotards—even

though some of the new ones are virtually irresistible.

■ Buy good equipment when you know you'll use it—otherwise rent until you're sure this is the sport for you.

■ Start simple. A $5 jump rope (Don't buy the kind they sell at the dime store for kids—it won't be heavy enough) can give you all the exercise you need and last a lifetime. Make sure your jump rope has ball-bearing handles.

■ Comparison-shop—Sears, Penney's and many discount outlets sell the clothes and equipment you need. If you don't need expert advice in picking out what you need, you probably don't need to buy at one of the more expensive pro shops. Also shop department-store sales, end-of-season sales and garage sales for equipment.

■ Good shoes are a must. I couldn't believe the difference they made in my stamina. The proper shoes really make me feel secure; they grab the surface and ensure that I don't fall, and protect my feet from the pounding of constant exercise.

MOTIVATION

If you need motivation, go to a health spa or club for a day and look at all the bodies around you. It is frightening to see what can happen to neglected flesh. Go to the beach and look at the passing parade. In twenty or thirty years, do you want to look like that? I thought not. So it's time to get crackin'.

My Work-Off plan is not a big weight-loss scheme or a quick shape-up for summer. It is an *everyday plan for the rest of your life* which maintains your weight while it *tightens* and *tones* the body. The Work-Off includes three parts:

1. Six-Day-a-Week Exercise Plan (set your own schedule)
2. Three-Times-a-Week Aerobic Sport for 12–15 minutes
3. Sunday Times

The regular exercise plan is simple and is based on the many classes I have gone to at various studios all over the country.

■ I don't believe in doing the exercises to music unless you're in a class; at home I think you should concentrate on counting.

■ If you miss a day's exercise, be careful the next day and go slower. Don't jump ahead, but continue a steady buildup. The more time you miss, the further back you have to go to start over.

■ Try not to miss a day, because it's easy to get out of the habit; a day becomes a month. Remember what you looked like before you got back into shape and use that mental image to motivate yourself.

■ Remember, before you go to bed at night, put your exercise mat and weights out so they are staring at you in the morning. If they're in the closet, you'll think of an excuse to leave them there.

■ Also remember, some days will be easier than others. One of the beauties of this program is that you can do just a little if it's all you can handle that day. You will go through phases.

■ If you have neglected your figure, the first year is to undo neglect and build strength, the second to tone and shape, the third to perfect and refine isolated areas. I know it sounds grim, but it does take a lot of work.

For your aerobic exercise or sport, you can probably find an activity you like that will give your heart the regular workout it needs. You can ride a bike or a stationary bicycle, jump rope (No matter what the weather, you can always jump. That's one of my favorites;

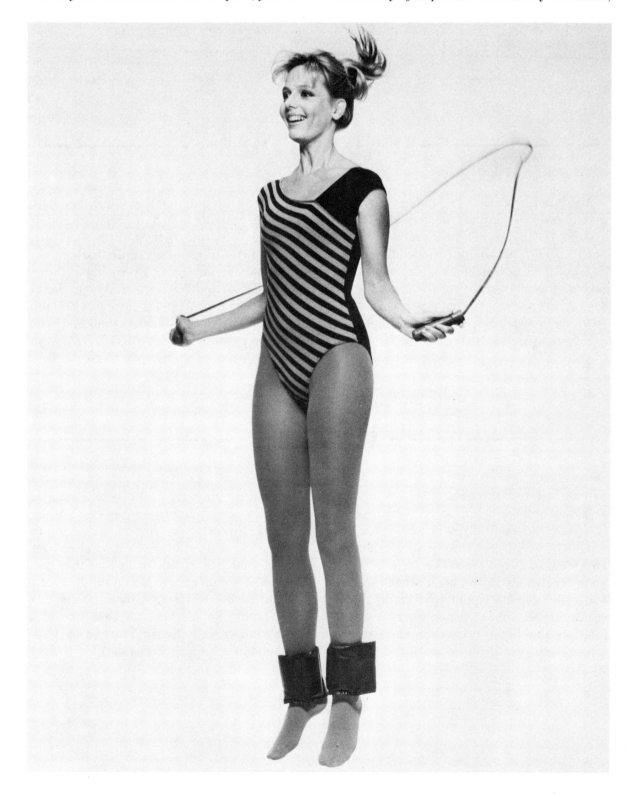

you can do a lot for your heart rate and stamina in a short time this way), jog, use a mini-trampoline, swim or even take a class. (I'm not that big on classes, as you already know, but I must admit that I do love to go to Lotte Berk method classes—it's the only controlled class I've found. I also swim laps in my backyard pool during the summer.)

This is in *addition* to my Work-Off. You need to have twelve to fifteen minutes of aerobic exercise at least three times a week. Continue the pace steadily; do not yo-yo. Don't tease your heart. My Work-Off is a strengthening and agility-building program. Aerobic exercise is for your heart. *You must do BOTH.*

SUNDAY TIMES

My Sunday Times are simple. I used to give myself the day off for casual relaxing around the house. Then I realized that I could still do everything I wanted to on Sunday and *feel* as if I had the day off. I was lazy and casual—*with my weights attached to my ankles!* Now on Sunday, when I dress—which is usually in something simple like a jogging suit—I just attach a 2½-pound weight to each ankle and go about my business. The weights look like cuffs on my jogging suit—no one notices them—and I'm doing a little extra for my figure without any extra work on my part! Even simple things like going up and down stairs give my legs a great workout! (You can cover the weights with fabric to coordinate with your clothes if you're very conscious of them.)

WEIGHTS

I use a set of 2½-pound weights for my exercises because I am pretty advanced in this plan. (After all, I did develop it for myself.) The beginner, however, should not use any weights at all. Once you have built up your repetitions to the point when you are ready for weights (when you can do 100 of each exercise *without* them, you're ready to take on the lightest weights), begin with 1-pounders (you'll be using two of them); then when you reach 100 of everything, go on to 2-pound weights, and so on. You can buy weights at any sporting-goods or discount store. I like the kind with Velcro backing so you can attach them to either your ankles or wrists easily. If you don't want to spend the money or want to experiment before laying out dollars, fill two tube socks with sand or Kitty Litter. You can easily get a pound of sand into a tube sock.

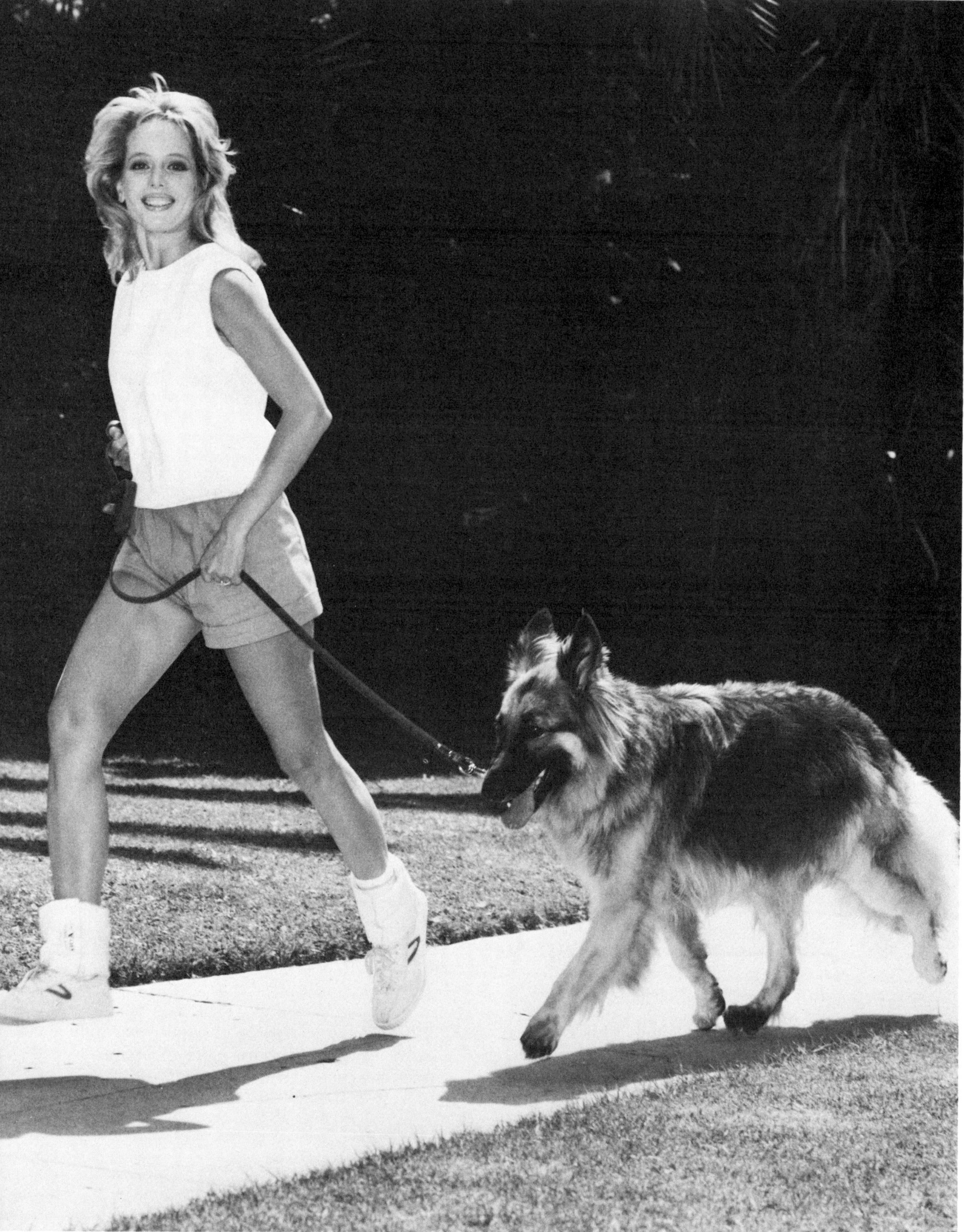

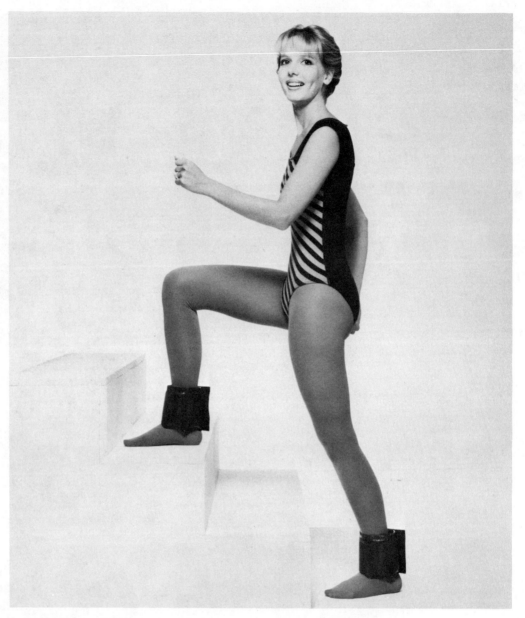

Too much weight is dangerous—it causes sprains and strains and makes you prone to more serious injury. I prefer high repetitions and low weights.

CHART YOUR PROGRESS

When you begin my Work-Off, measure yourself and write down the figures, either in this book or on a scrap of paper you can hide in a drawer. Measure yourself again every six months to see how you are doing. You should find that while you weigh the same, your figure has changed for the better. Don't expect miracle results in three weeks. It takes time.

Face your figure and do what you have to do to get it in shape. Look at yourself critically in a bikini—you'll always look better in a leotard and tights; the fabric holds you in and makes you look more shapely. Or check yourself naked and face facts!

WEIGHT: DATE:

measurements:	today	6 months	12 months	18 months	24 months
bust:					
waist:					
hips:					
upper arms:					
thighs: top thigh					
bottom thigh (above the knee)					
calves:					

As I said, this isn't a program for losing weight; it's for working off bumps and lumps and mounds and ripples and flab. It will help you get rid of five or ten pounds, but you'll need another method if you need to lose more than that. It will also help you gain strength. And I promise you, if you are faithful to the system (and yourself), you will see a tremendous change in your figure and your athletic abilities—in just six months. You'll also have the added bonus of more confidence and a feeling of well-being.

THE EXERCISE PLAN

The exercise plan is built on a series of repetitions, which are added to daily as you gain strength. The first time you do any of these exercises, do only the number of repetitions you can manage easily, even if it's *two.* The next day add another one or two, or whatever is comfortable. Add very slowly, and build up strength as you go. Never strain—build up over a period of time. This way there's no chance of injuring a muscle or having to stop because of hurting yourself. To actually change the shape of your body, you will need to do many repetitions (at least 100) and use weights. If you want to change flab to muscle, keep on counting. If you only want to stretch your body and stay in prime shape, do the exercise without weights or keep your repetitions lower. It takes a long time and a lot of weight to actually re-mold your body shape.

Warm Up

1. Stretch It Out

Standing position. Bend over at the waist and let yourself droop forward with the weight of your torso pulling you over. You can touch your toes or the mat, or just stretch a little if you want to. Hold for a count of 10, then slowly straighten up again. Repeat.

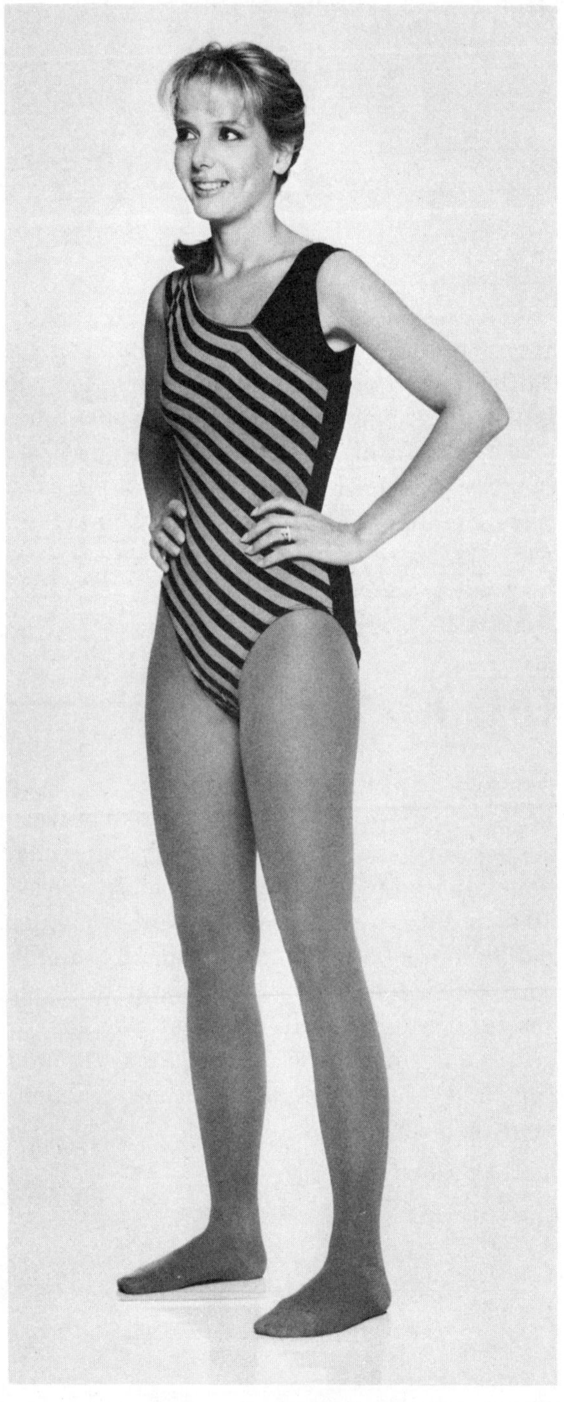

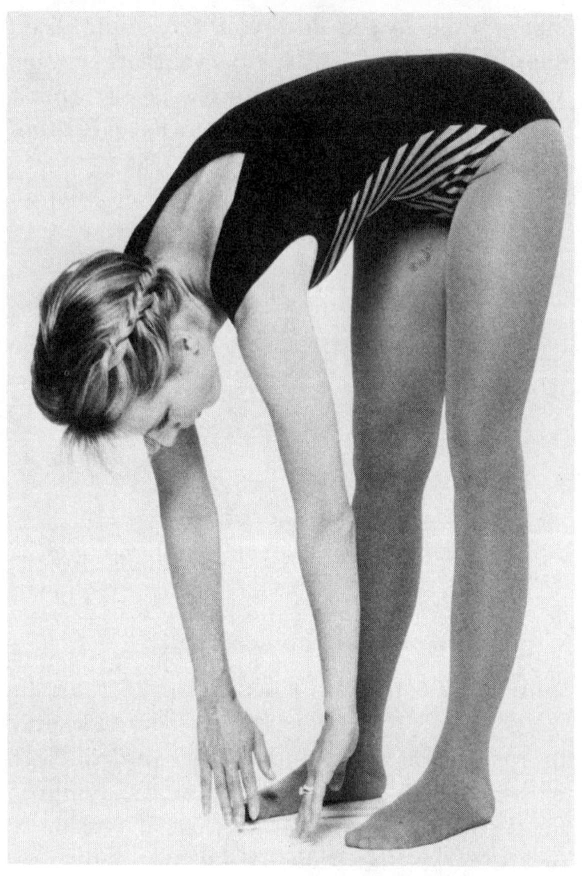

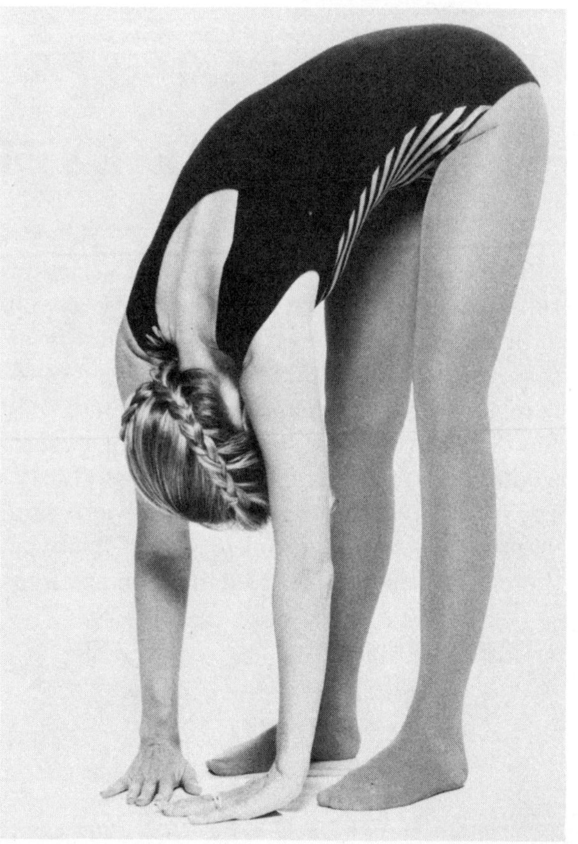

2. Stretch Up

Standing, reach for an apple that is overhead. Reach and grab, reach and grab. Do this a few times to warm up. (You do not have to count.)

3. Side-to-Side Stretch

Now bring your arm over your head and bend from side to side a few times, again to help you warm up. Bounce a little and pull gently on those tight muscles. No counting—this is just to get going.

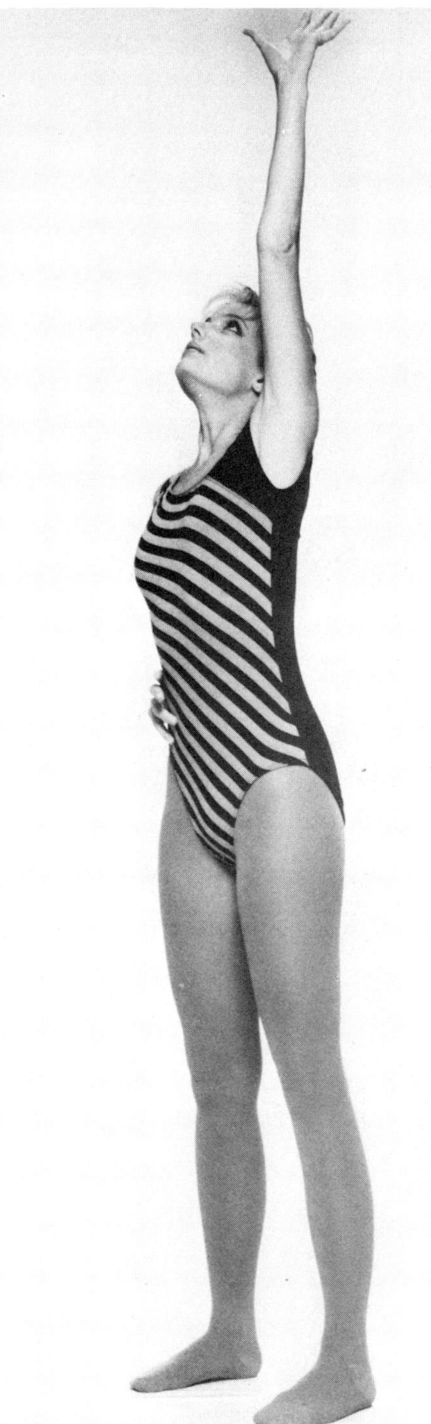

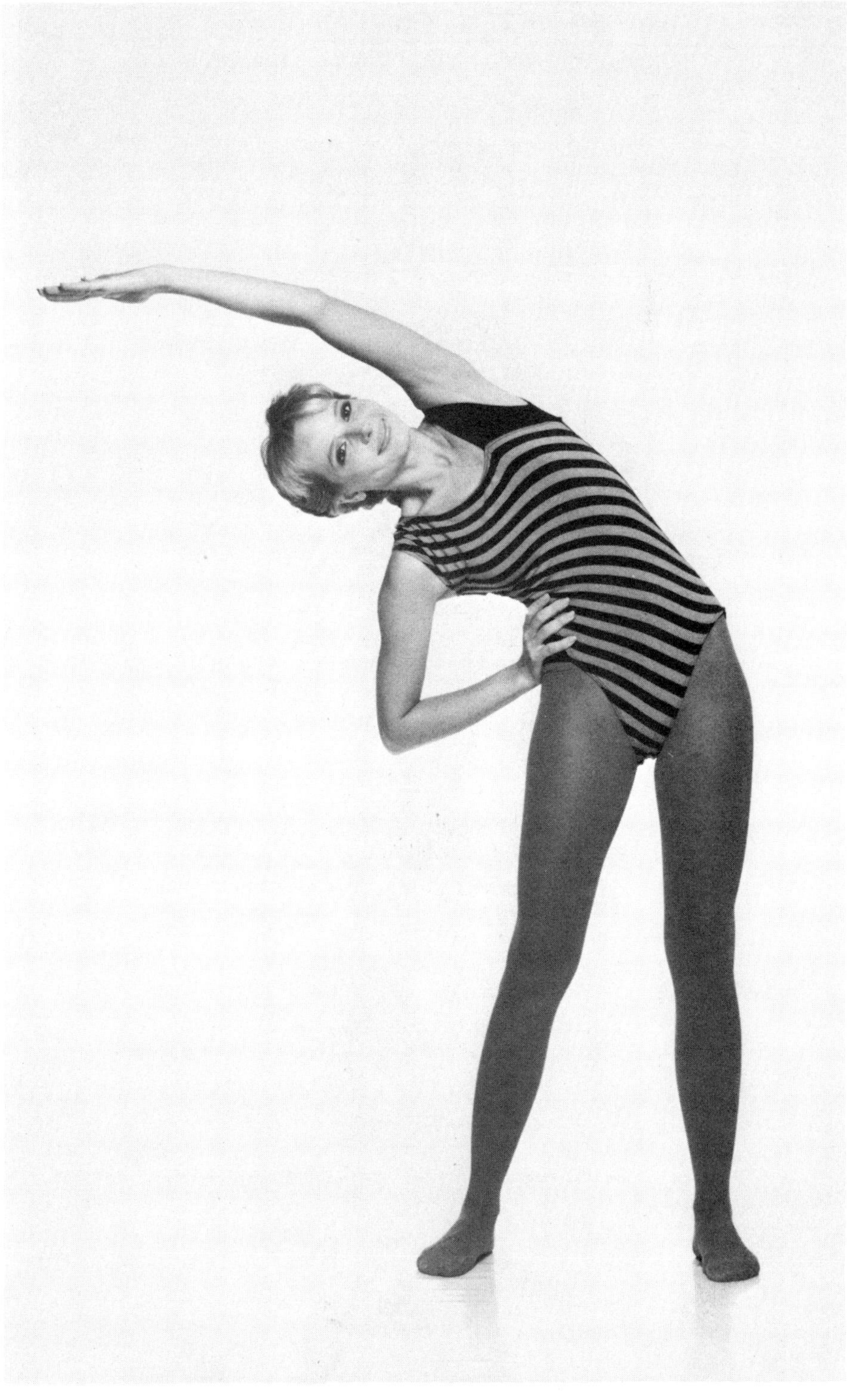

4. Jogging in Place

Stand with feet parallel, toes even with each other; place your hands on your waist as you lift feet one at a time. Beginning with small lifts, go higher and higher. Since it's so hard to count steps, time the jogging instead. Begin with one minute and work your way up to five. Since this is just a warm-up, you don't need to jog any longer than that.

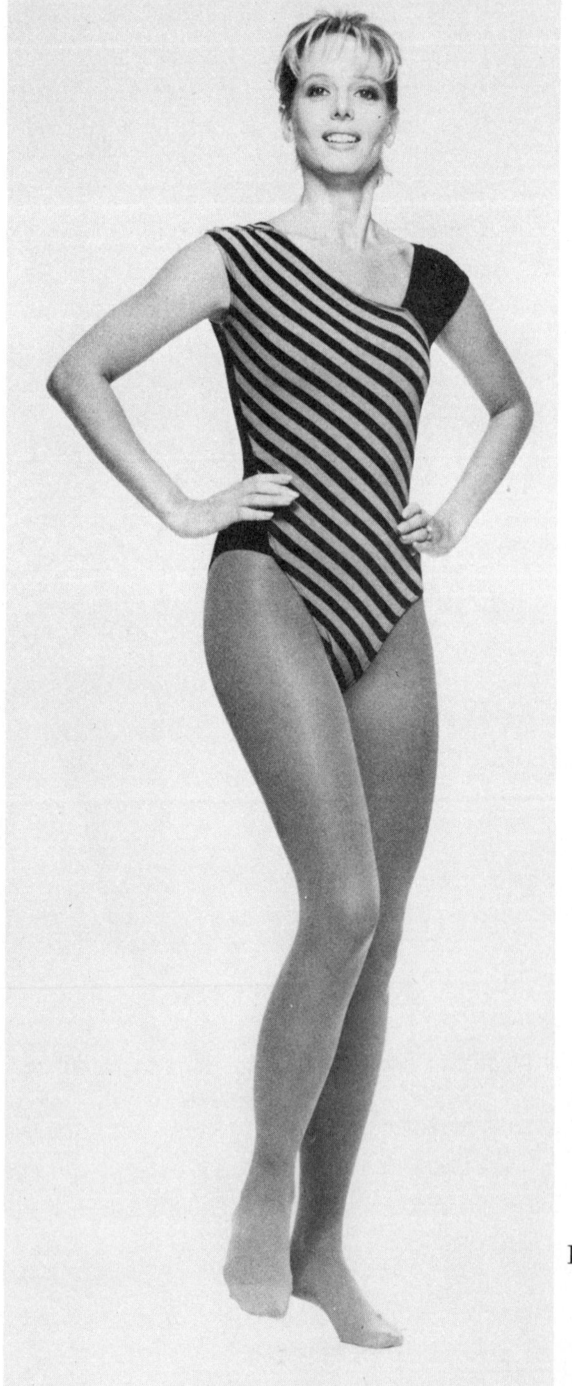

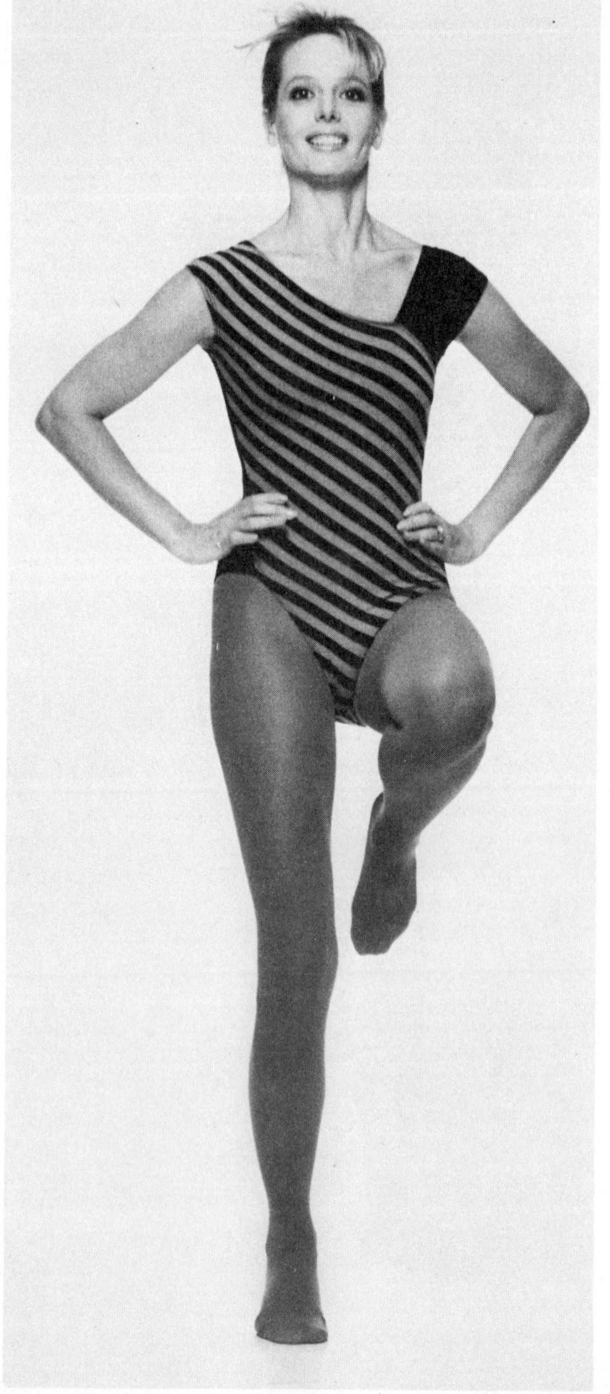

Okay, warmed up? You should be.

Never begin any exercise without warming up!

If you're ready for weights, this is when you attach them—or grip them. Weights go around the ankles for leg exercises, around the wrist or held for arm and torso exercises.

The count: Count out loud as you go. This will force you to breathe. (Many times you concentrate so hard that you forget to breathe.) Your goal is to reach 100. Remember, if you miss even one day or more of the Work-Off, go back to whatever number you can do *easily*. Don't push it—do stop before 100. Always build up slowly; never strain. If you start your Work-Off and find you aren't in the mood, do as much as you can stand anyway and then quit. Just do a little every day, no matter how much you'd like to skip it. When you have really built up strength, hold the extensions for several seconds before releasing.

Work-Off:

For exercises 1, 2, 3, 4 and 6 always keep your seat tight, your stomach in, shoulders down and back.

1. Forearm Curls: Stand on your mat with your feet apart and your arms down, hands forming fists (or gripping your weights) in front of your thighs with palms facing *up*. Your elbows should be slightly bent against your body, your back straight and shoulders back. Now bring the fists (or weights) up to your chest alternating right, left, right, left.

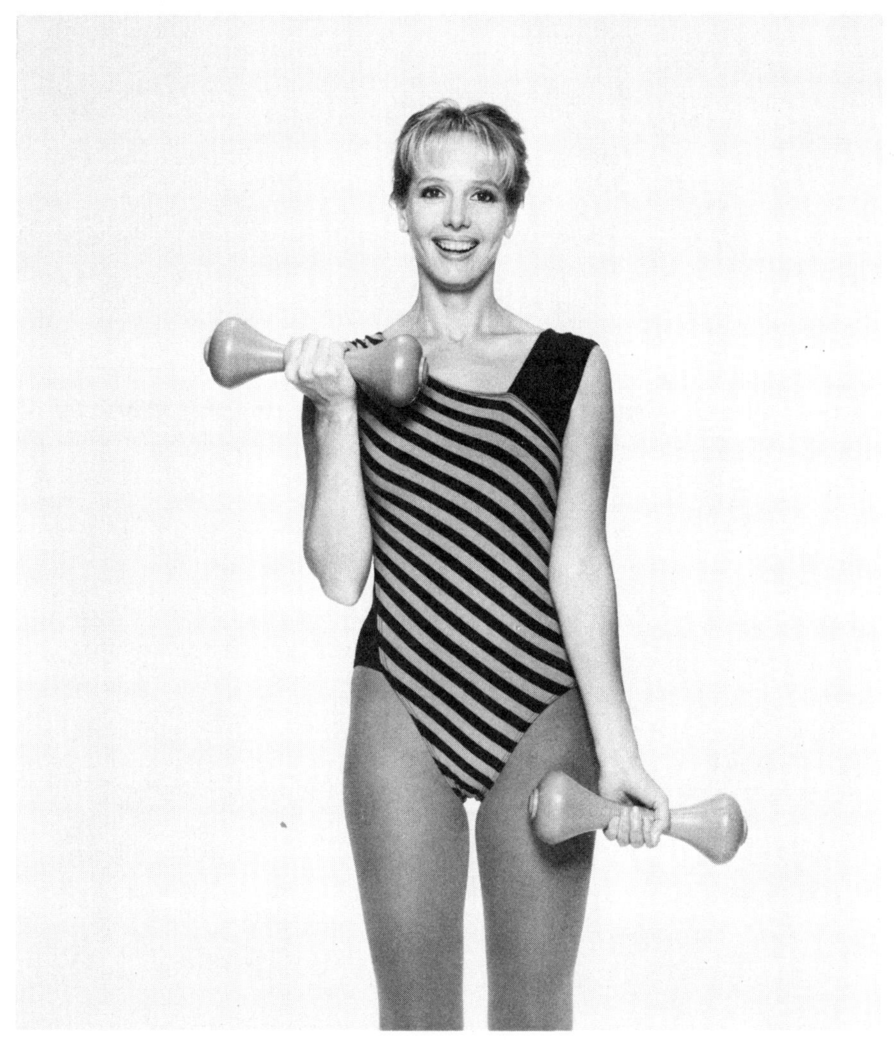

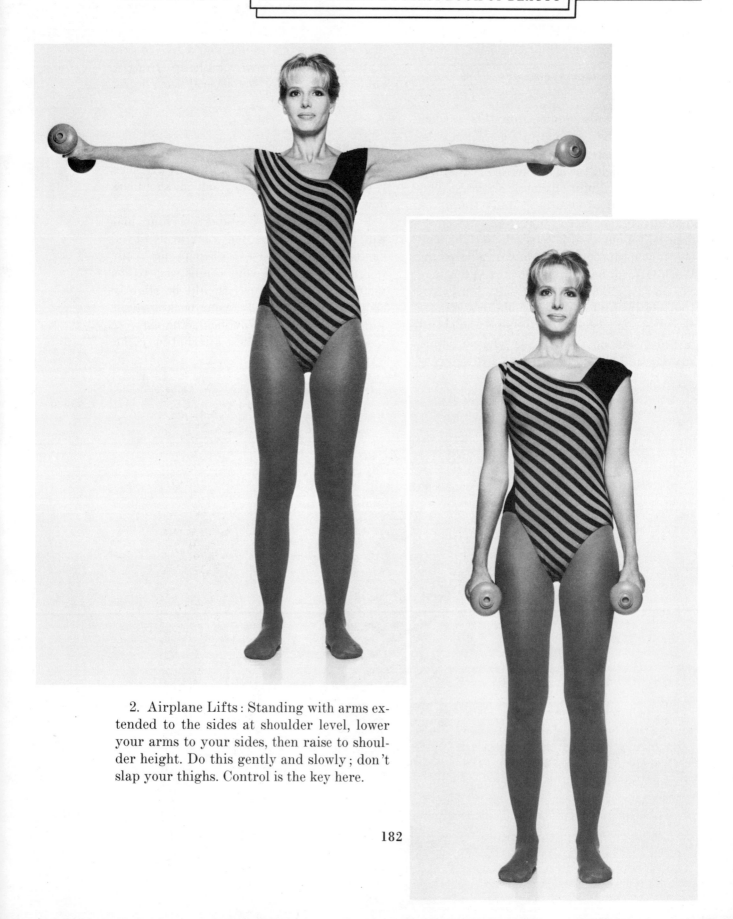

2. Airplane Lifts: Standing with arms extended to the sides at shoulder level, lower your arms to your sides, then raise to shoulder height. Do this gently and slowly; don't slap your thighs. Control is the key here.

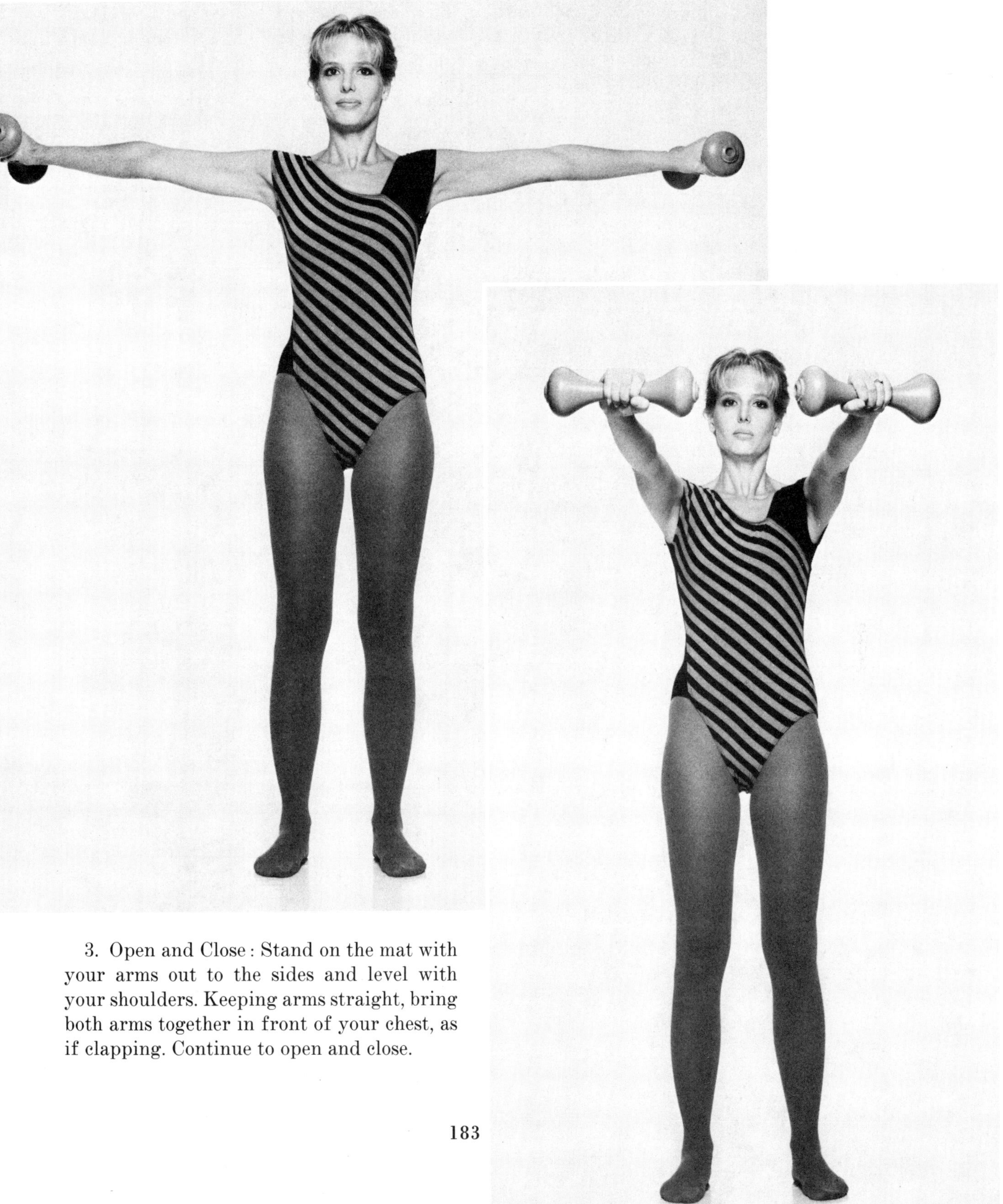

3. Open and Close: Stand on the mat with your arms out to the sides and level with your shoulders. Keeping arms straight, bring both arms together in front of your chest, as if clapping. Continue to open and close.

4. Criss-Cross: Standing position, with arms extended to the sides. Cross your left arm over your right in front of you at chest level. Open arms slightly to the sides again, then cross the right over the left. Don't swing your arms around. Continue in a scissoring motion.

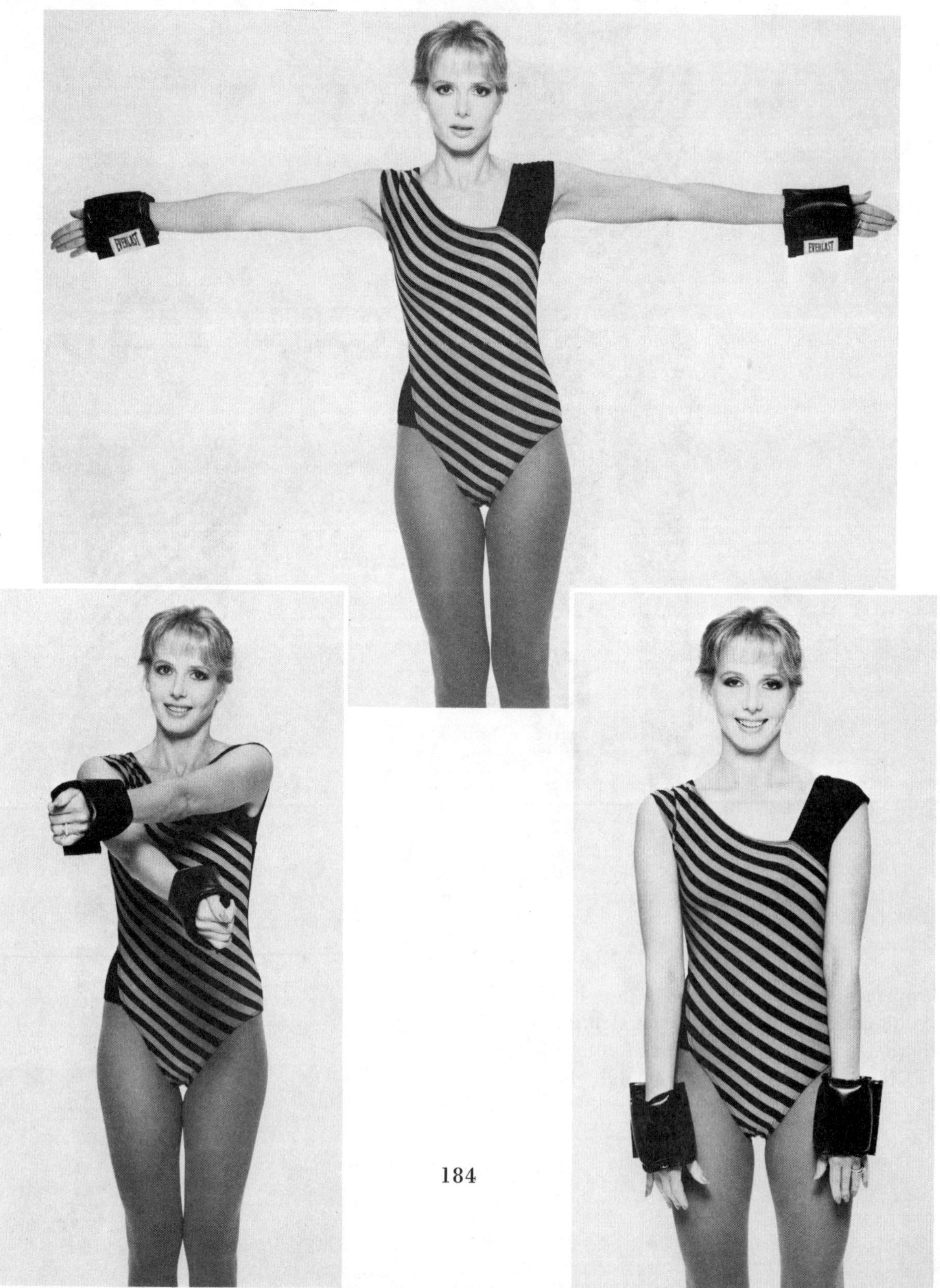

5. Arms Up: Start with both arms down, hands in front of thighs. Bring your right arm *straight* up over your head, in an arc in front of you. Lower it to your side, then repeat with your left arm. Continue, alternating sides.

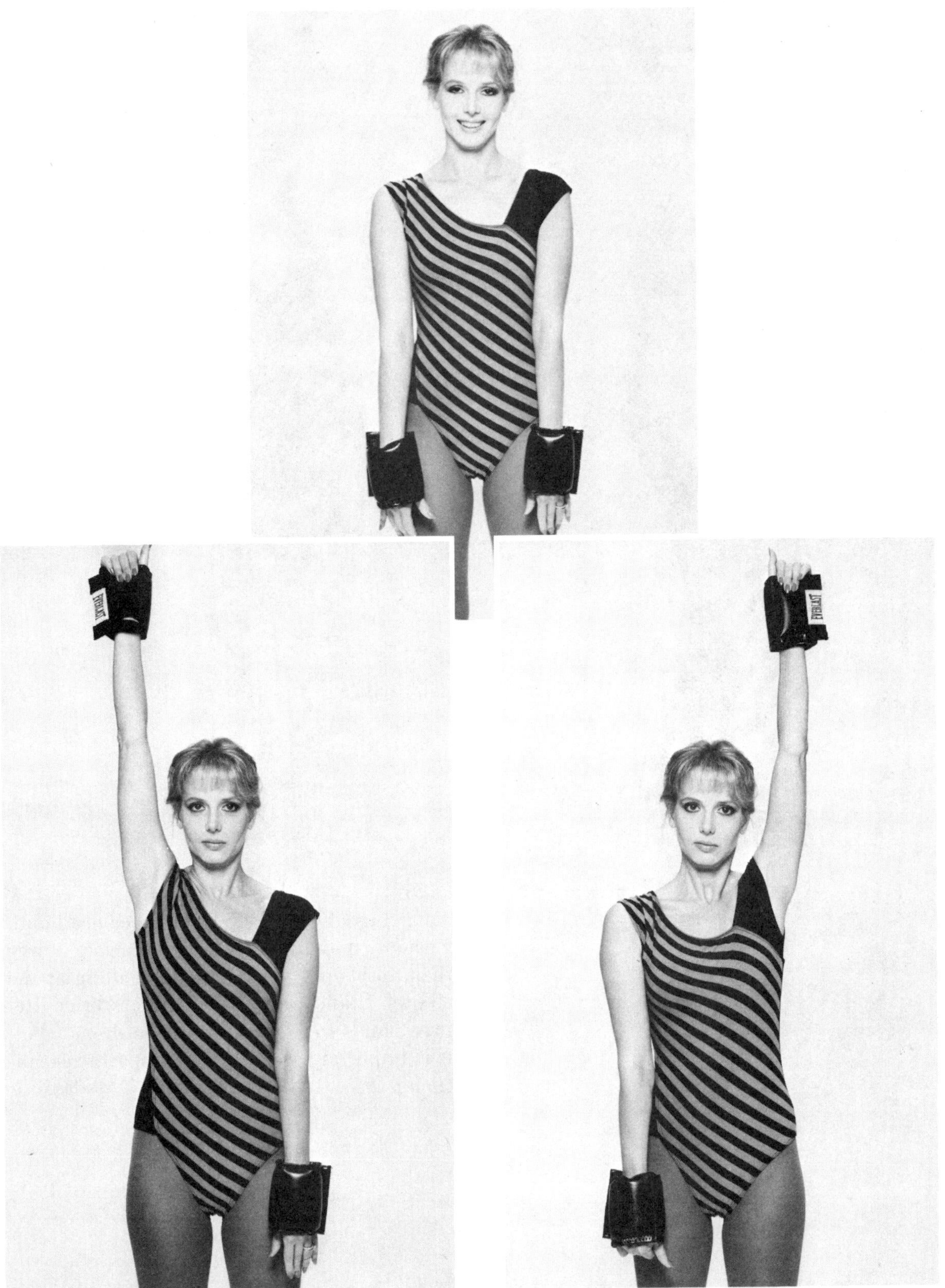

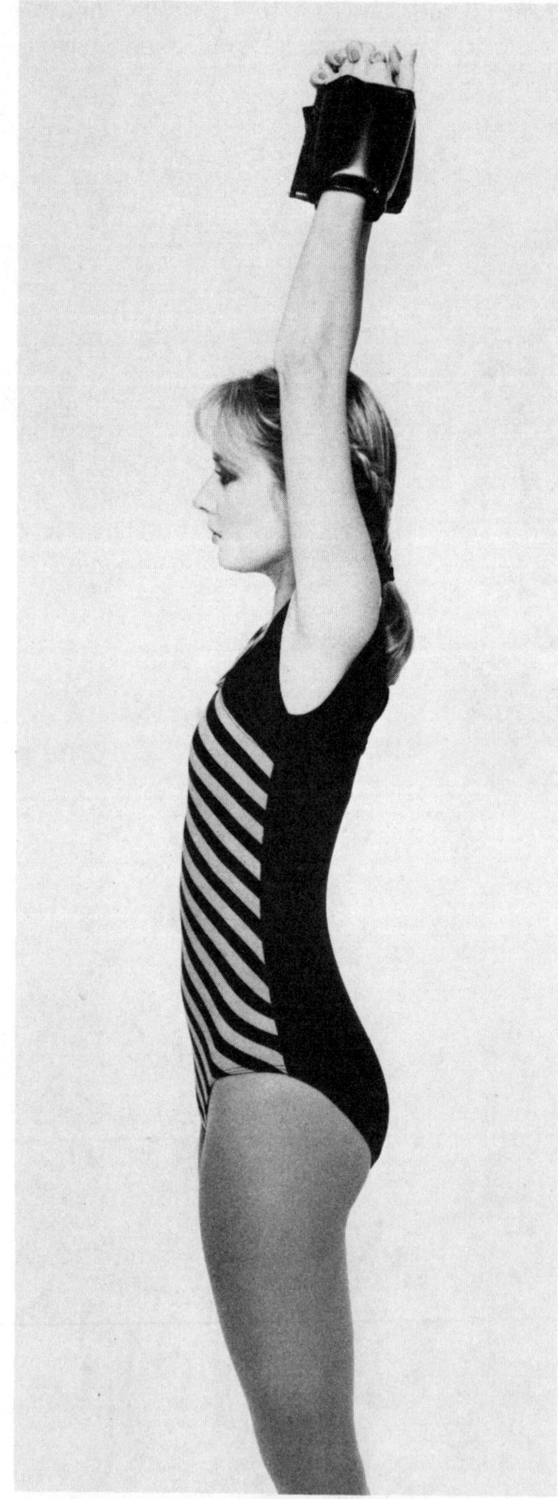

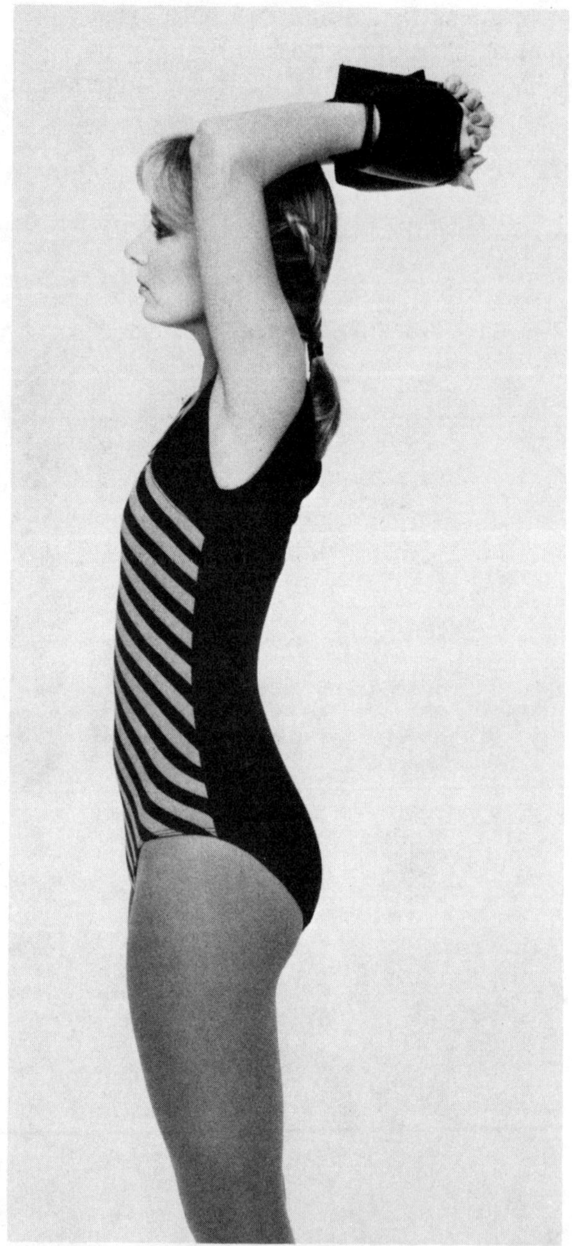

6. Hand Ups: Clasp hands over head and, without moving your upper arms, lower them to behind your neck by bending at the elbows. Stand tall with shoulders back. Return hands to overhead position. Remember, it is important to keep your upper arms stationary!

7. Side to Side: Stand with legs apart and arms at your sides. Bend at the waist as far to the right as you can, sliding your right hand down your thigh for maximum stretch. Come back to upright position and repeat to the left. Keep the shoulders back, the tummy in, seat tight, and don't lean forward.

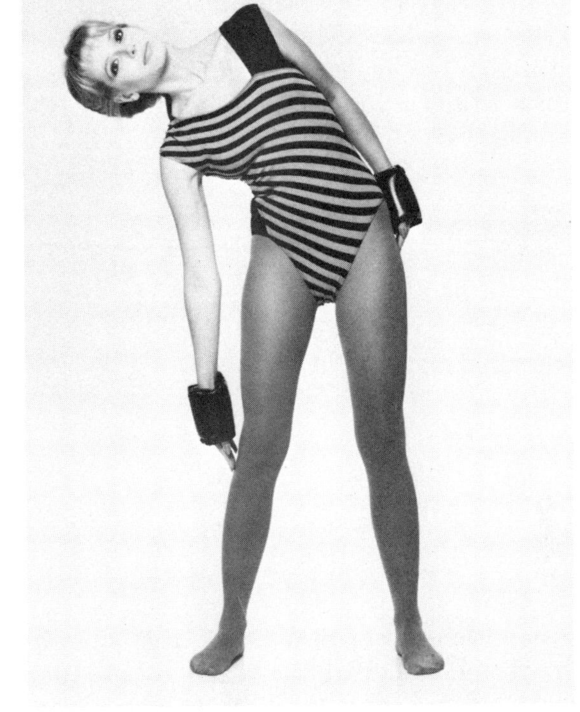

Variation: Do the same exercise with arms extended straight overhead, keeping arms close to your ears as you bend from side to side.

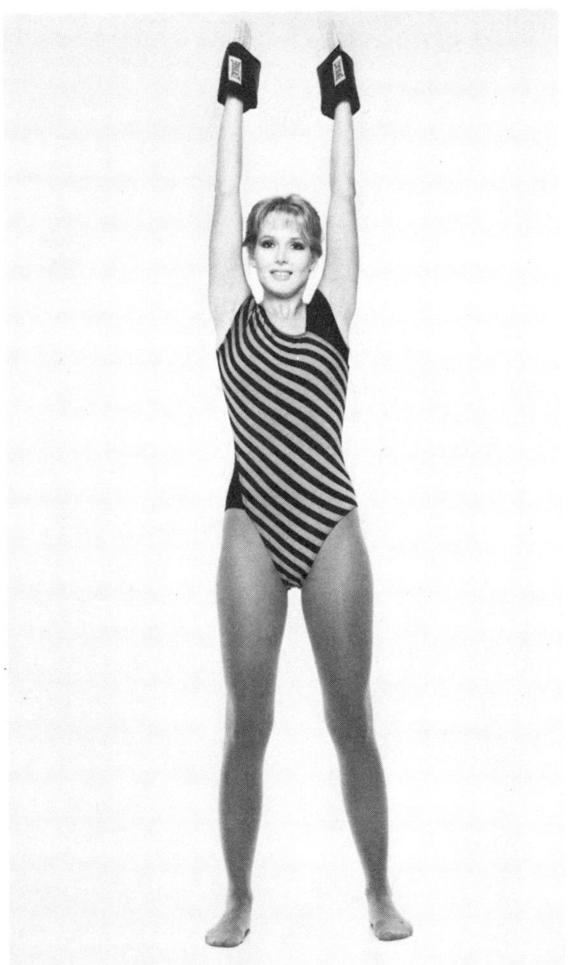

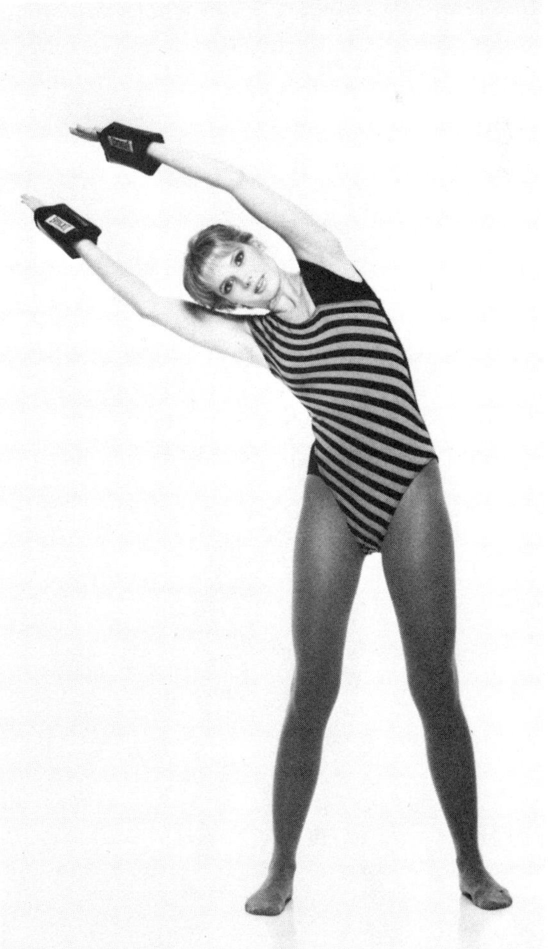

8. Side Rises: Stand with legs apart and arms at sides, shoulders back and back straight. Lower one arm as low as you can drop it along your side while you raise the opposite arm to the waist. Alternate sides.

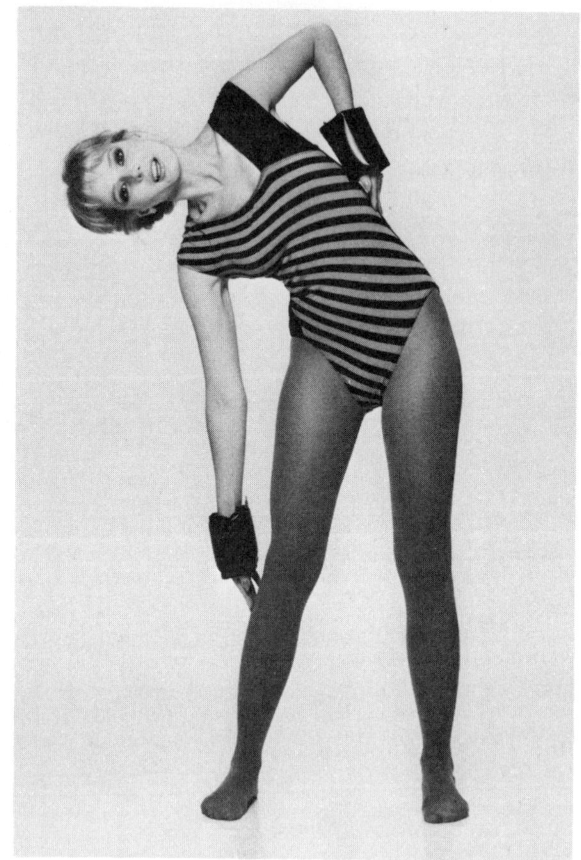

9. Reach Over: Stand with legs slightly apart and hands at the waist. Reach your right arm up and over your head to the left and lean left. Stretch your whole side from underarm to waist, as well as the waist itself. Then alternate sides.

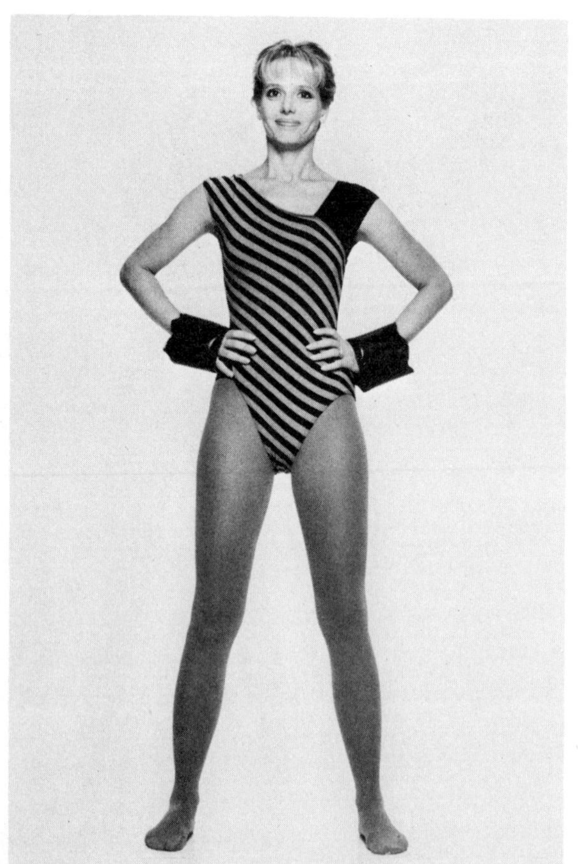

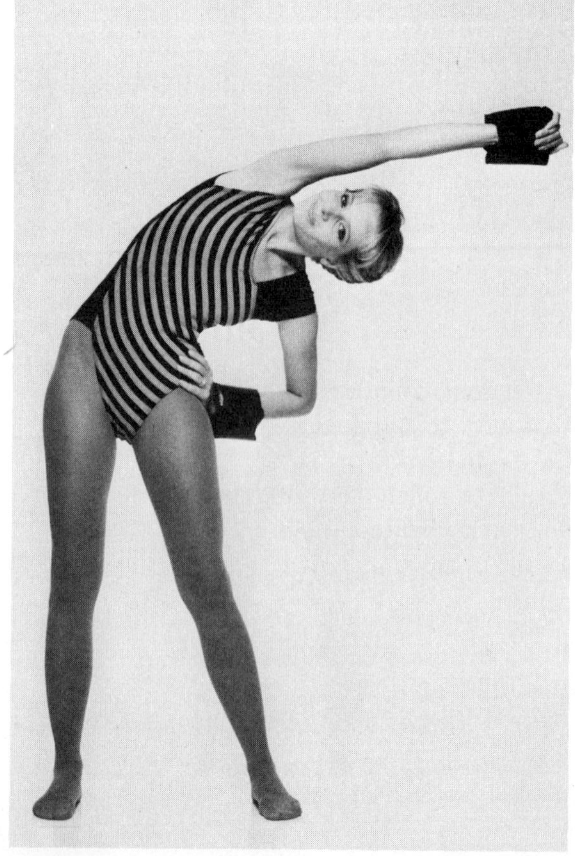

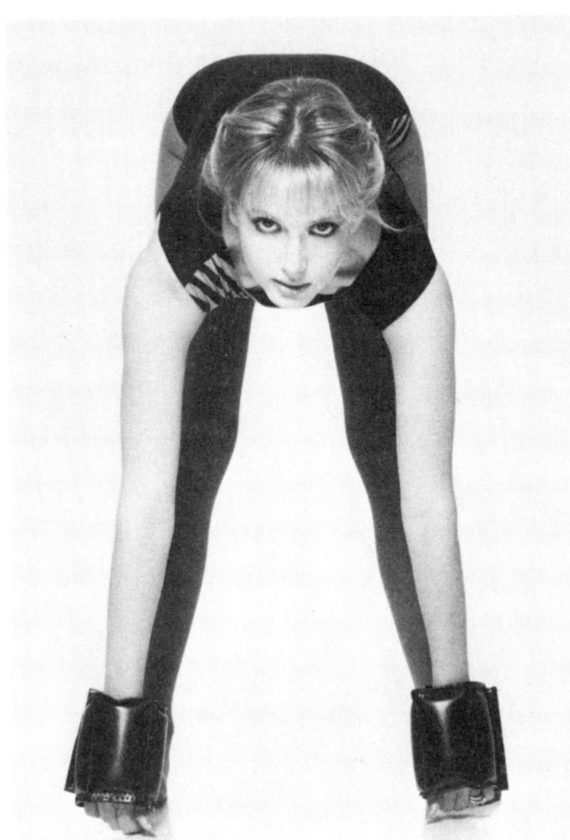

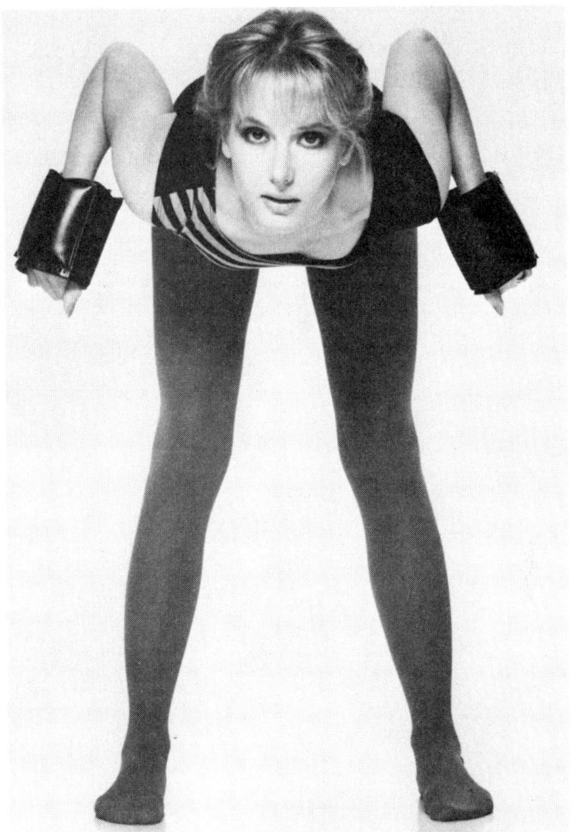

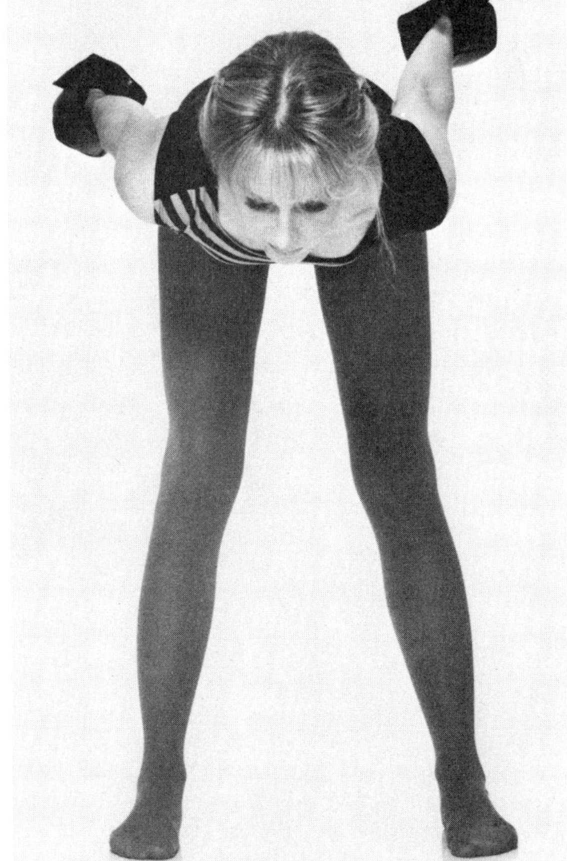

10. Arm Benders: Bend forward at the hips with feet apart and back flat. Drop your hands to the floor. Then raise elbows and hands to touch your rib cage. Now extend your arms behind you, parallel to your back, to work the upper arm. Stand upright and repeat.

Now sit down on the mat (not the floor!). Attach weights to ankles if you are ready for them.

11. Upper Abdominal Lifts: Lying down on your mat, cross your legs at the ankles and bring knees to chest with arms crossed over your chest. Lift your upper body slightly and release. Here again, it's important to hold the tummy in and to breathe out as you lift.

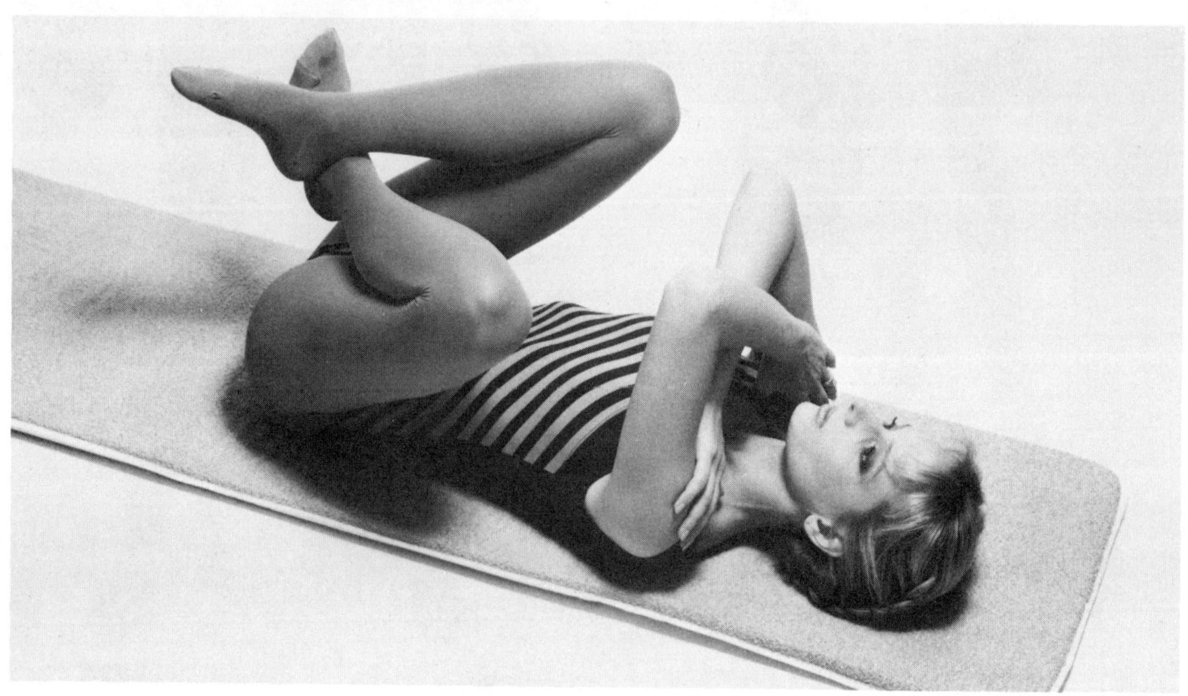

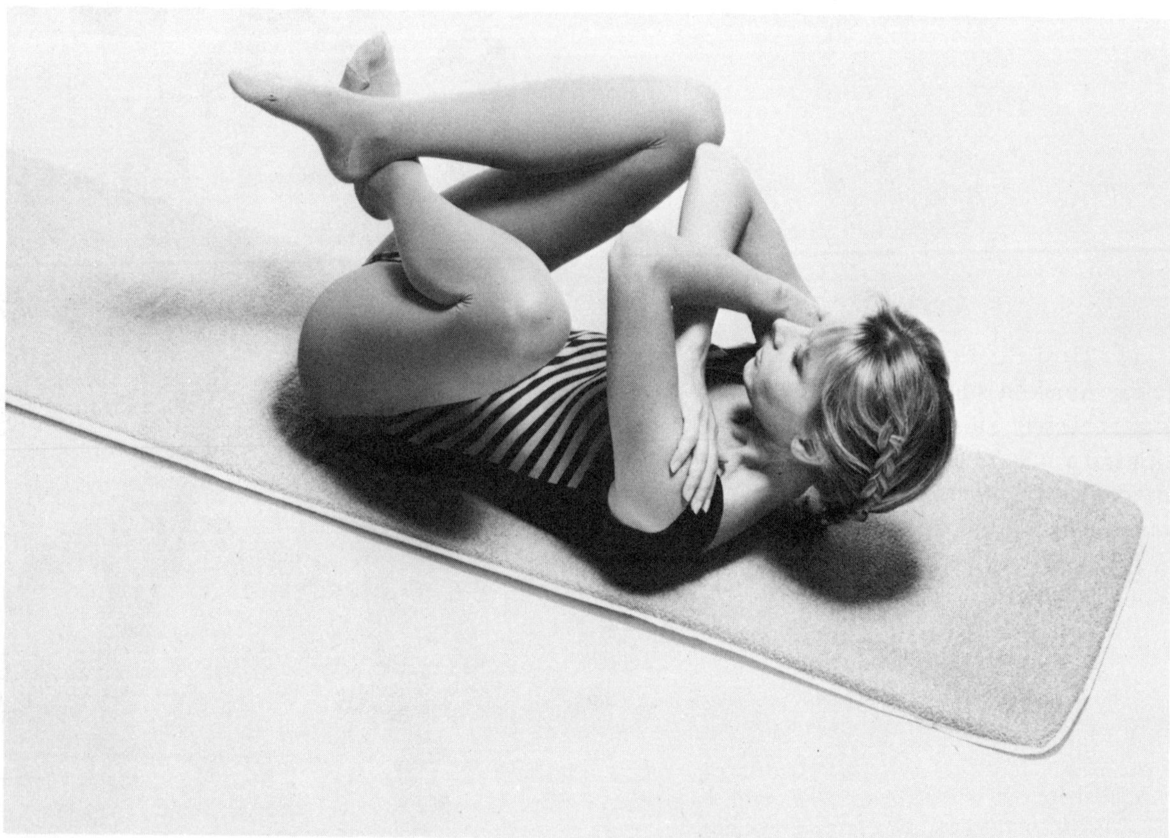

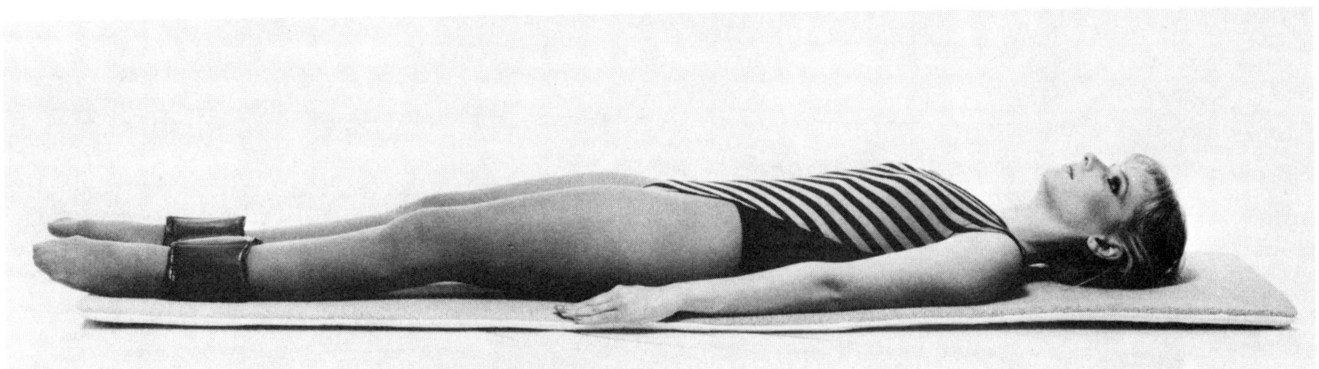

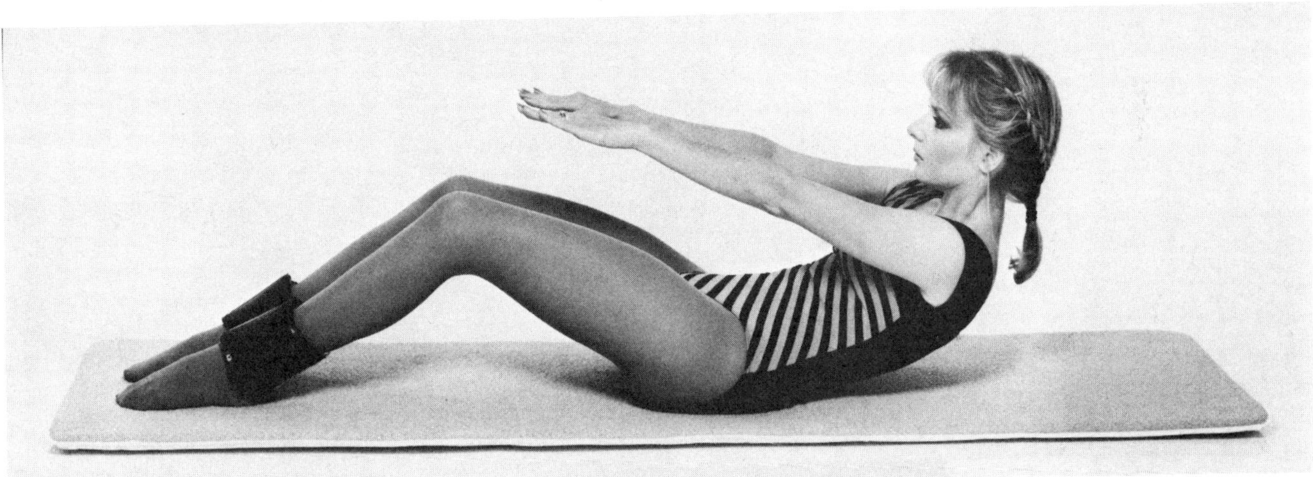

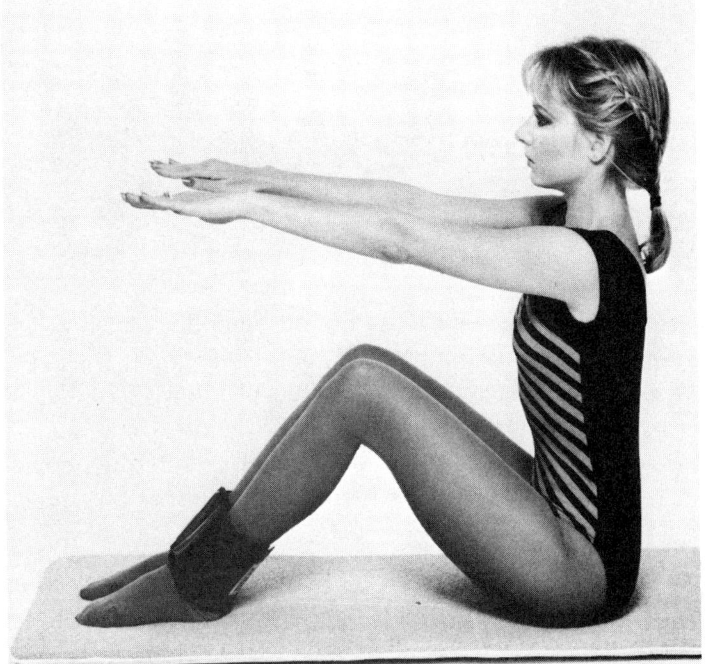

12. Mini Sit-Ups: Lie down on your back with your knees bent, tummy in and buttocks tight. Slowly raise your head and shoulders toward your knees and sit up, arms extended in front of you for balance. Release slowly. Exhale as you sit up, and hold your stomach in, otherwise you can get a bigger tummy! Release slowly.

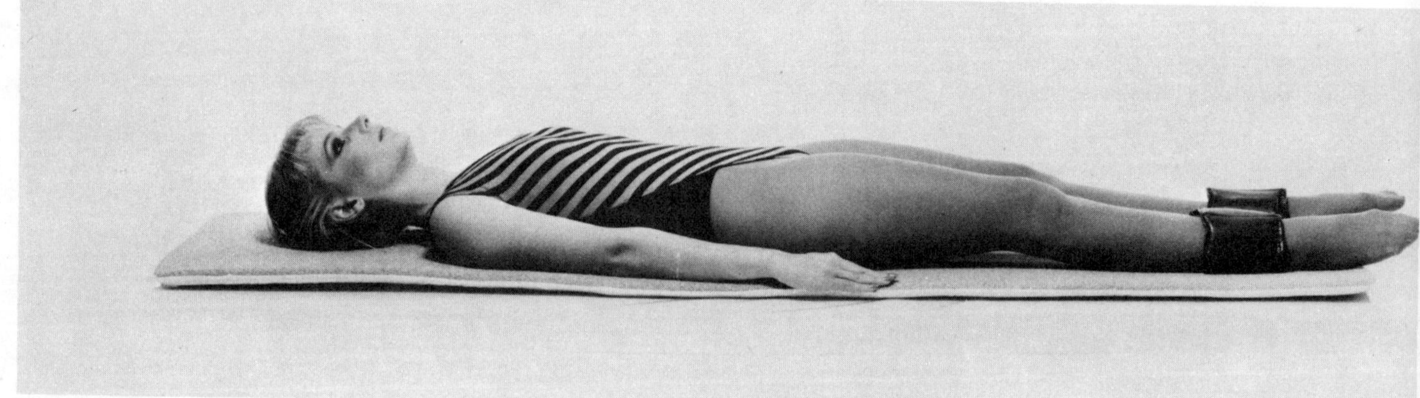

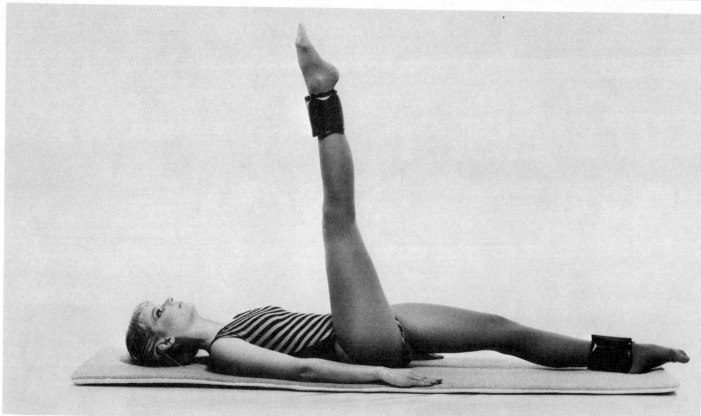

13. Leg-Ups: Lie on your back with your legs extended. Lift one leg straight up, toes pointed, until it is perpendicular to floor. Lower it to floor and lift again. Do as many as you can with one leg before starting on the other, keeping both legs straight at all times.

14. Double-Ups: Now bring both knees up to your chest; then slowly extend both legs up together. Release, bringing knees back to your chest, keeping toes pointed. Do only 20–30 at the most!

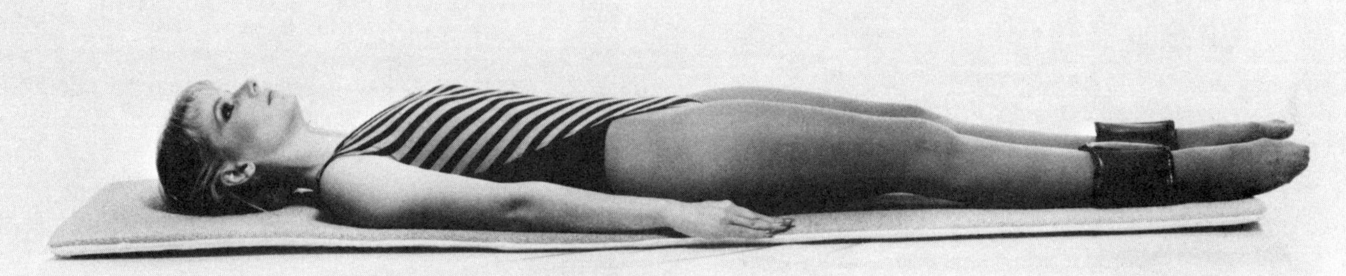

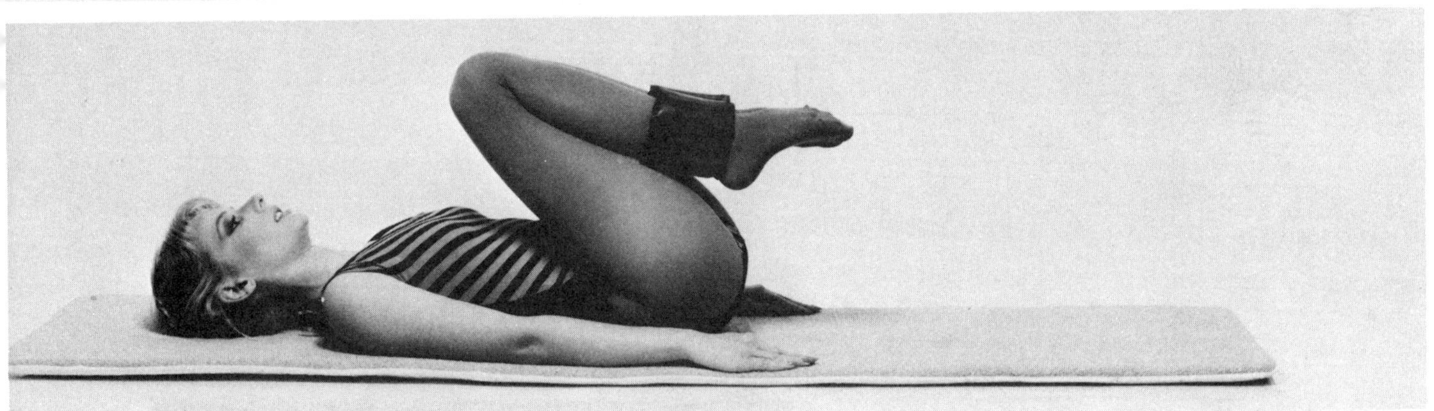

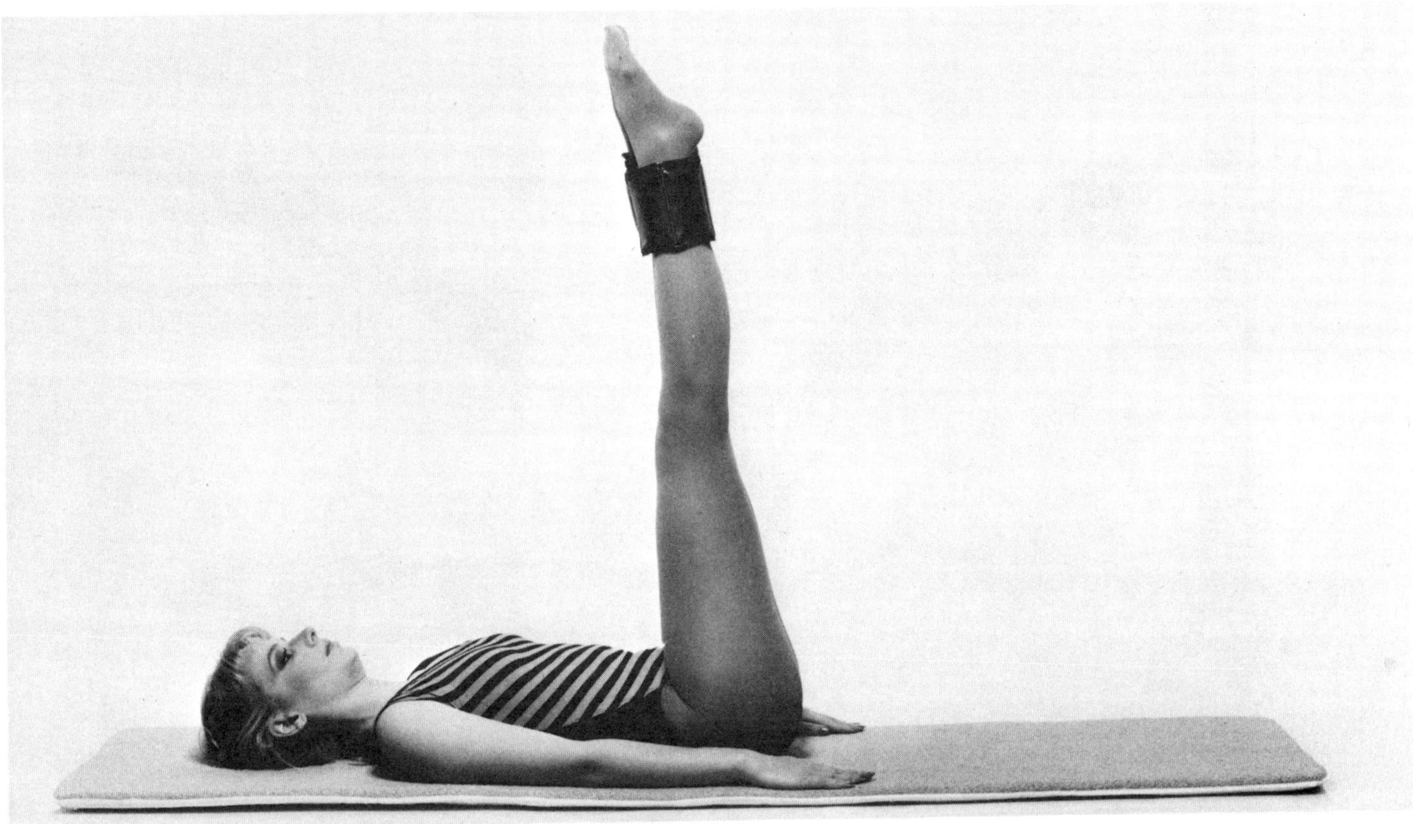

15. Scissors: On your back, extend your legs together, straight up. Open legs, feet flexed or pointed, in a wide V. Bring them together again firmly.

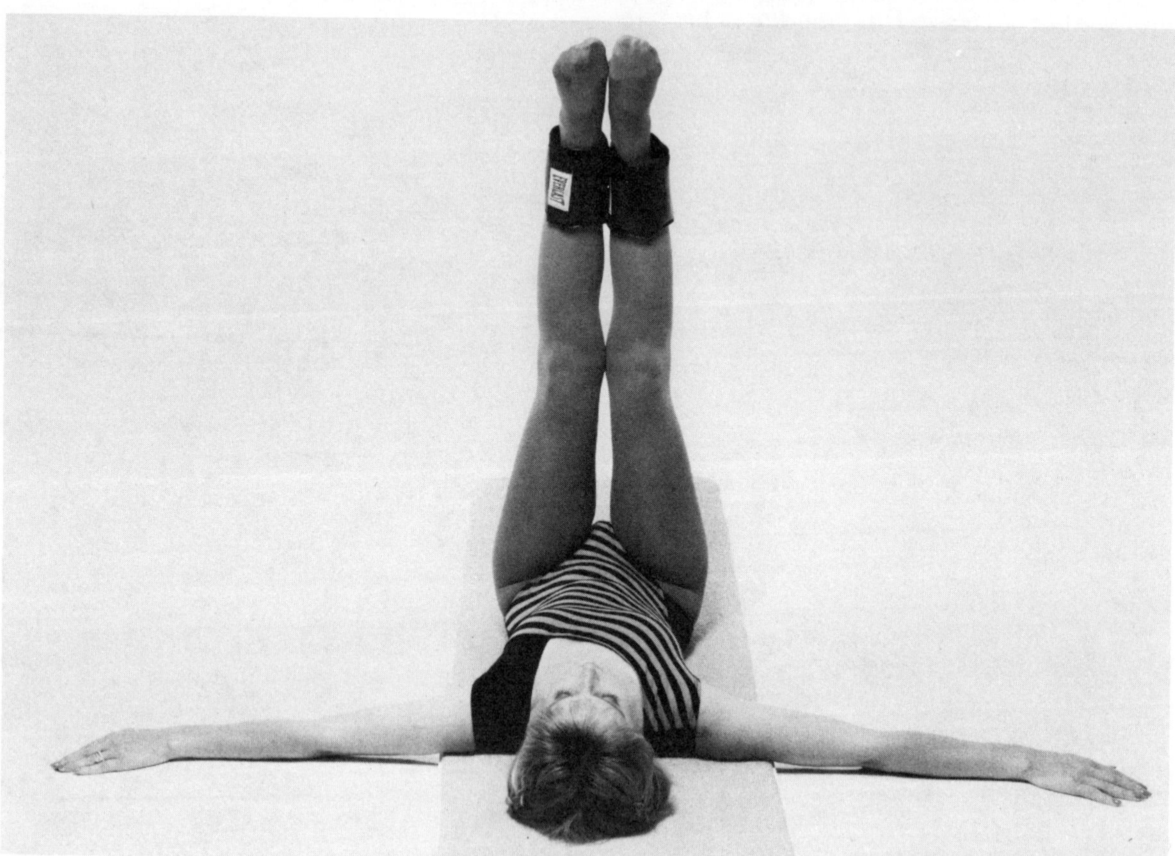

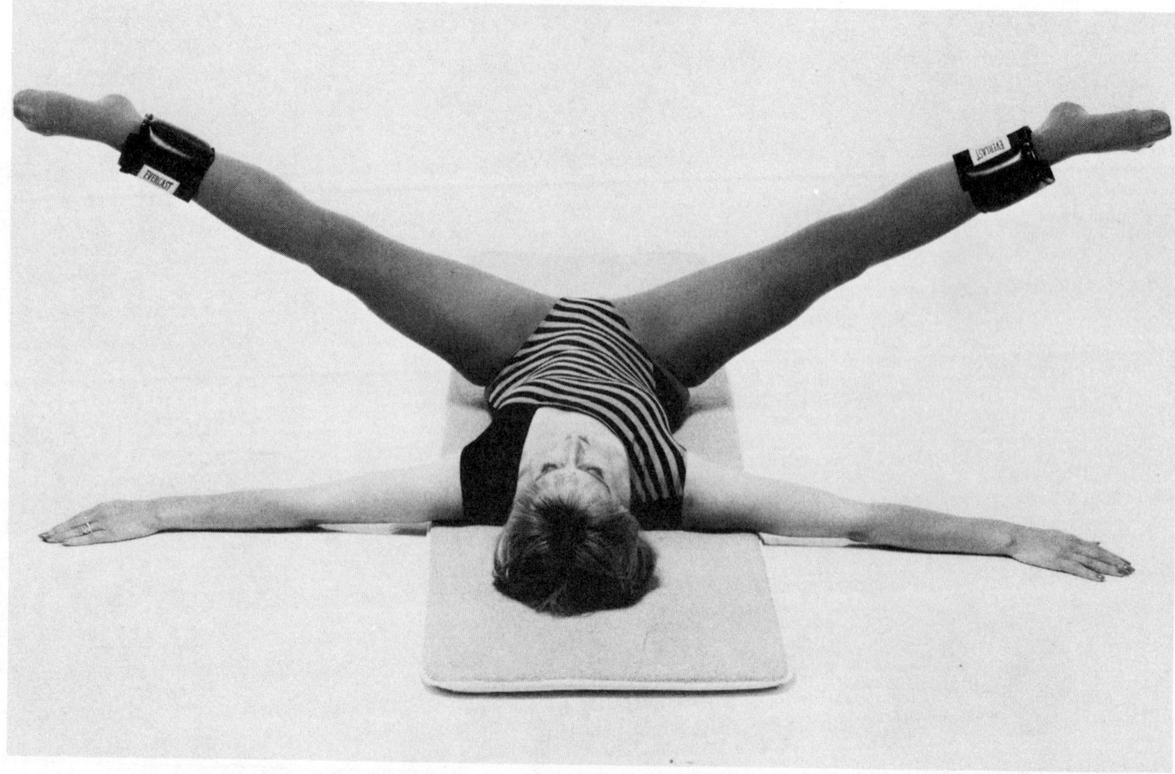

Variation: After opening legs bring together again, this time crossing the right leg under the left. Open about 2 feet apart, then scissor the left under the right.

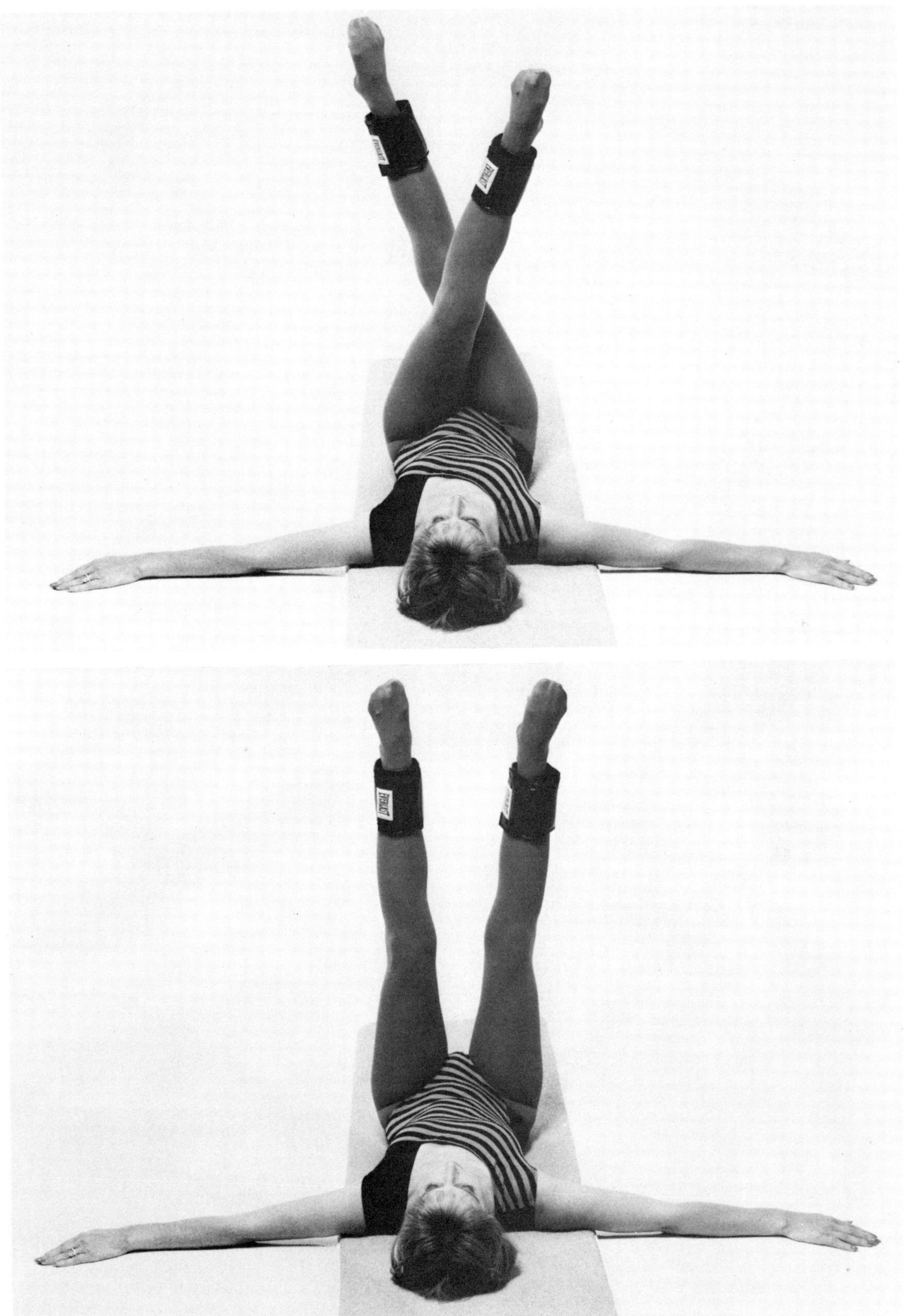

16. Leg Lifts: Turn onto your side, shoulders back, head up. With foot flexed, raise the top leg about 6 inches, then lower. Repeat as many times as possible, working up to 100 repetitions eventually. Next raise your leg higher (about 2 feet from the floor) and lower, repeating up to 100 times per side. Finally, lift as high as you can, and lower. Do

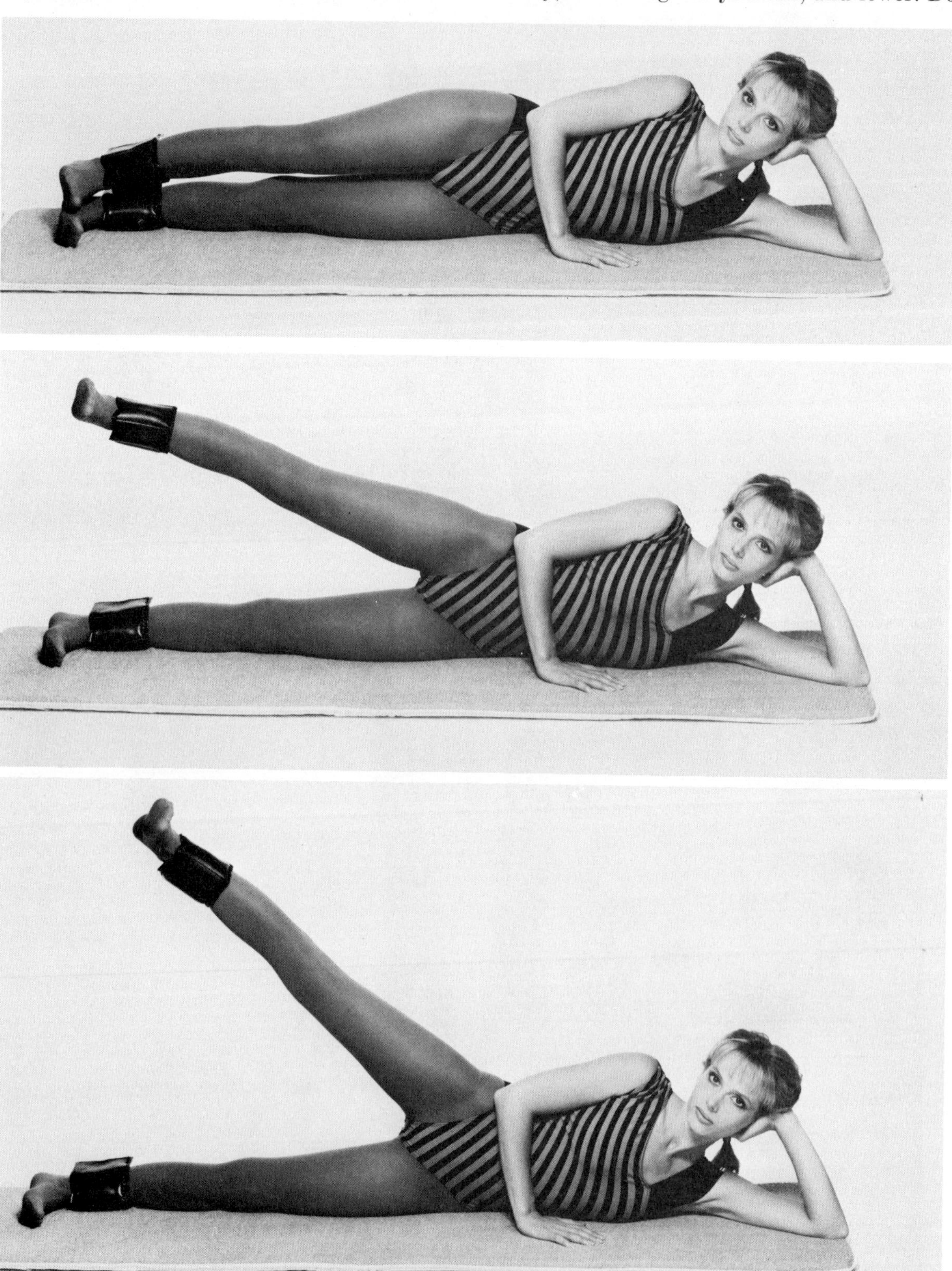

100 if you can! Be sure to keep your body aligned—hips, shoulders, knees—throughout. Complete all 3 levels on one side, then turn over.

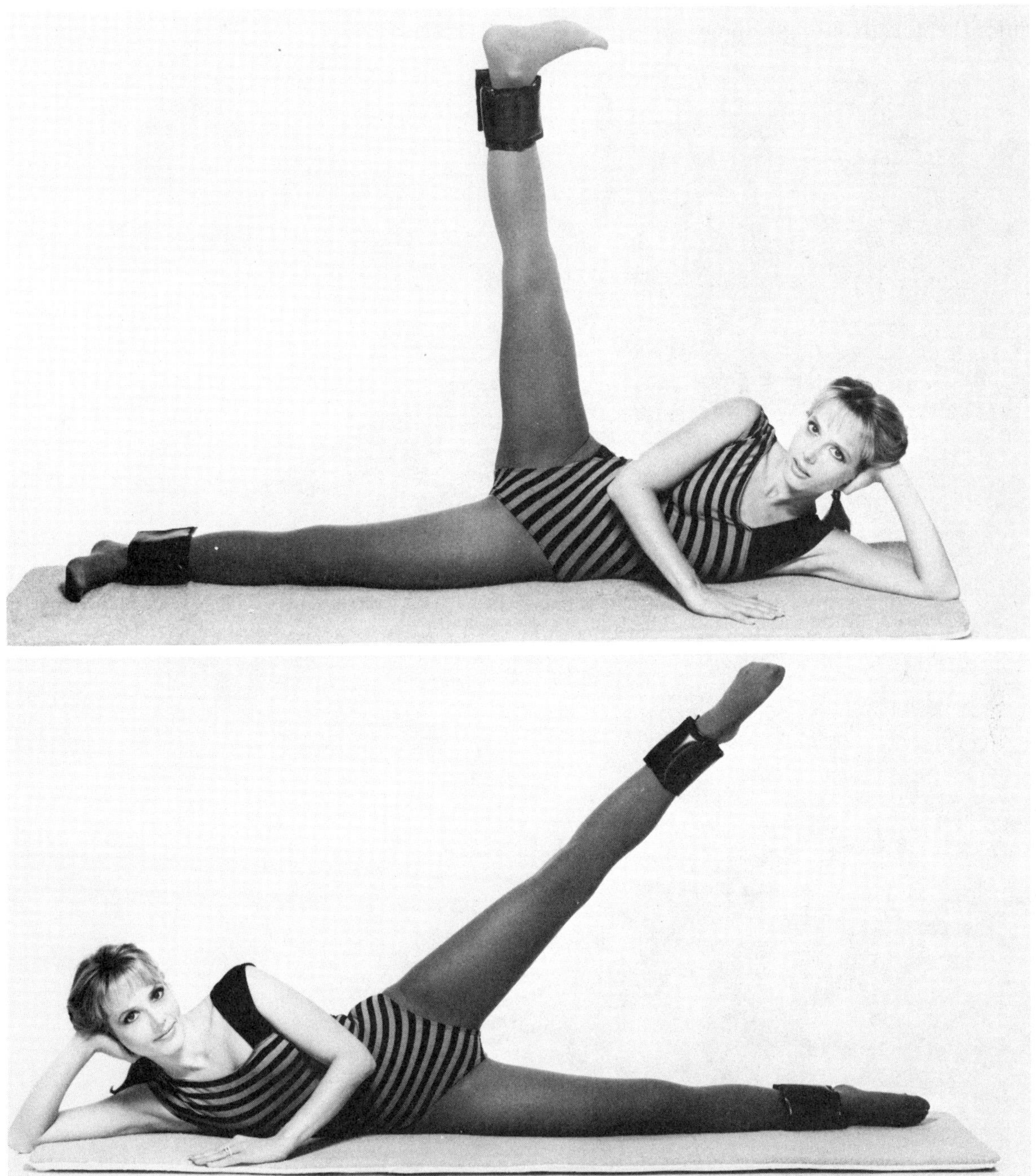

Variation: On alternate days, repeat as above, with toes *pointed,* knees facing the ceiling.

17. Buttocks Tucks: Lie on your back with knees bent and feet flat on the mat. Keeping shoulders on the mat, raise your buttocks into the air. Holding tummy in, lift and squeeze seat and release 10 times. This exercise should be done in sets of 10 (10 sets equals 100 repetitions).

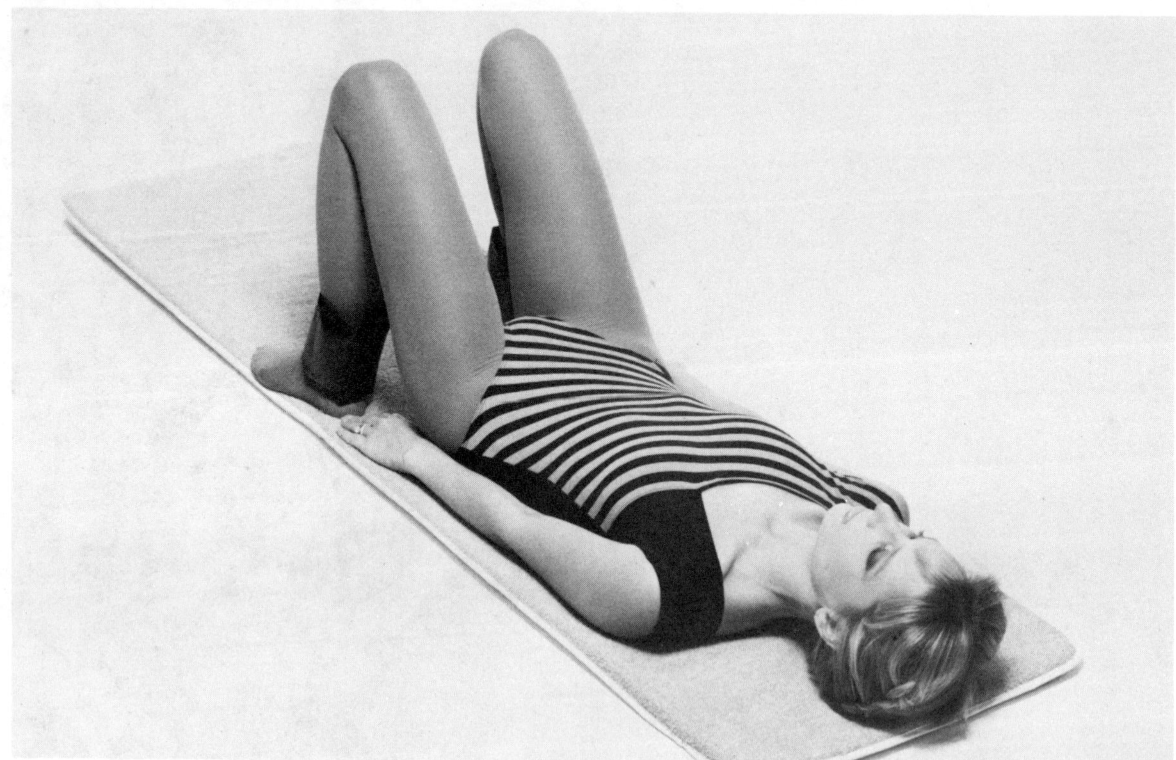

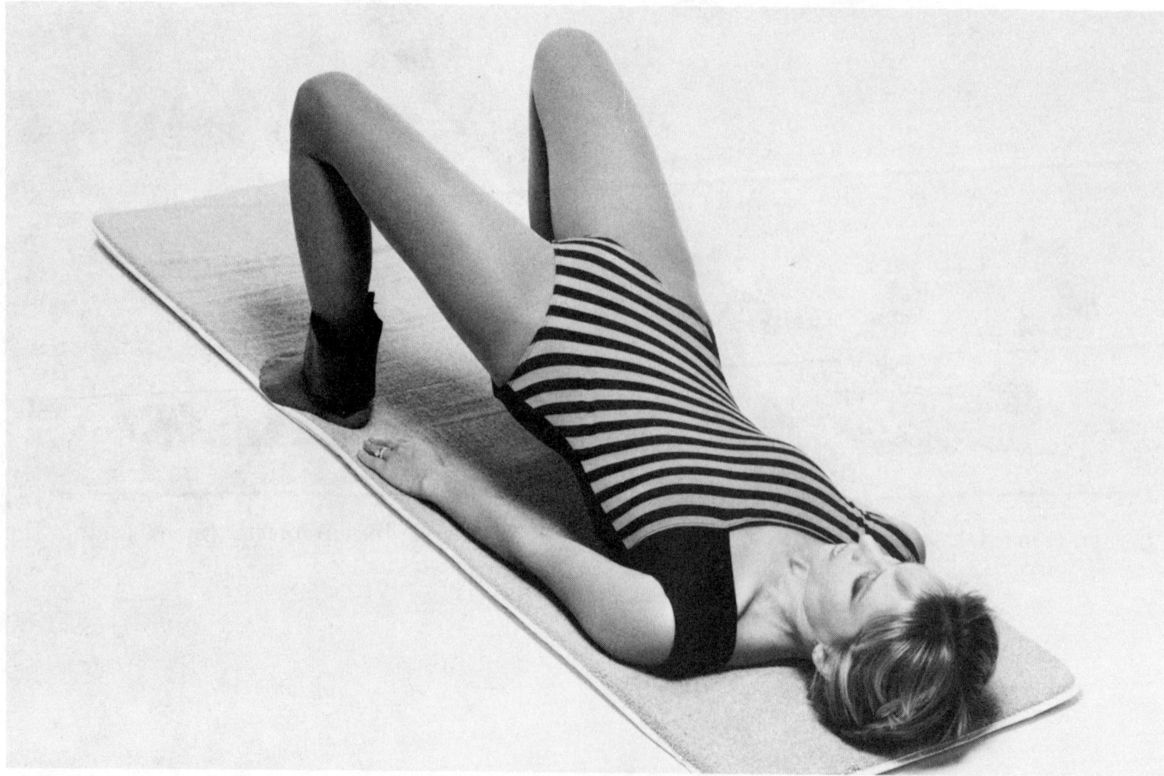

Variations: Do the same exercise with heels raised and your weight distributed on the balls of your feet and shoulders. Open and close your knees as you continue to tuck and release.

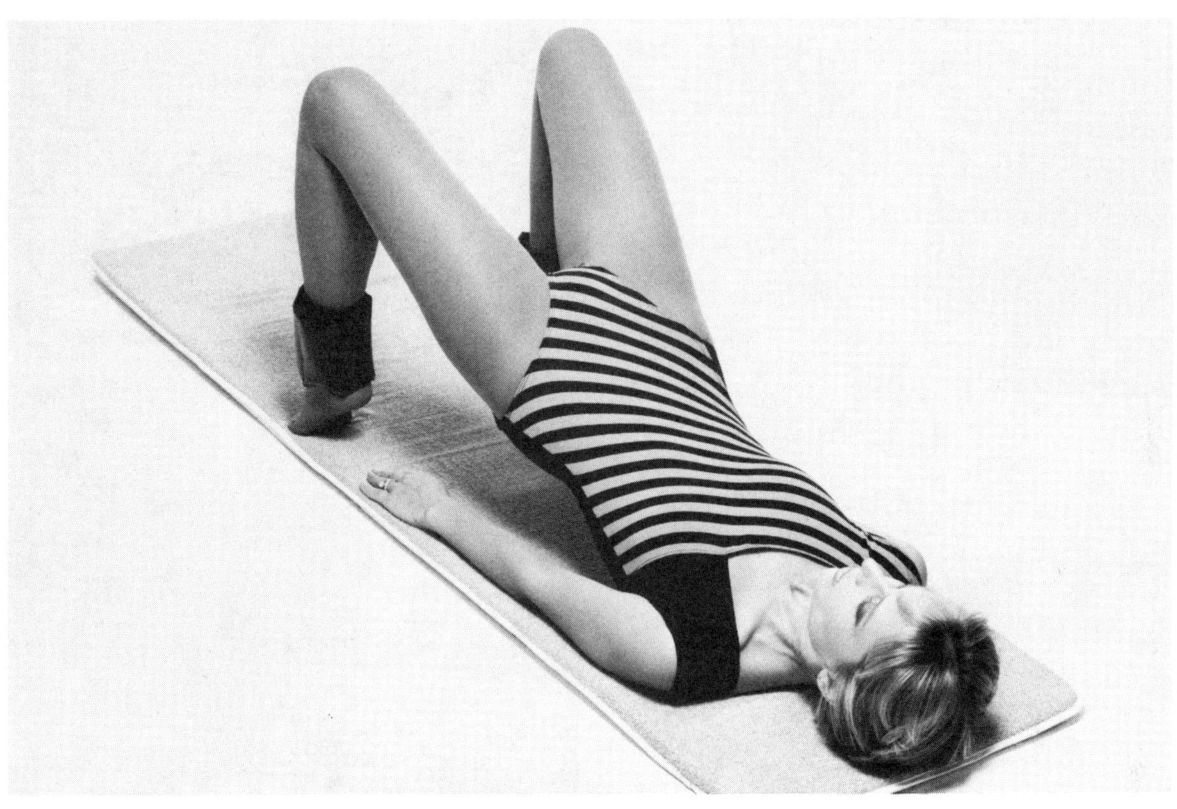

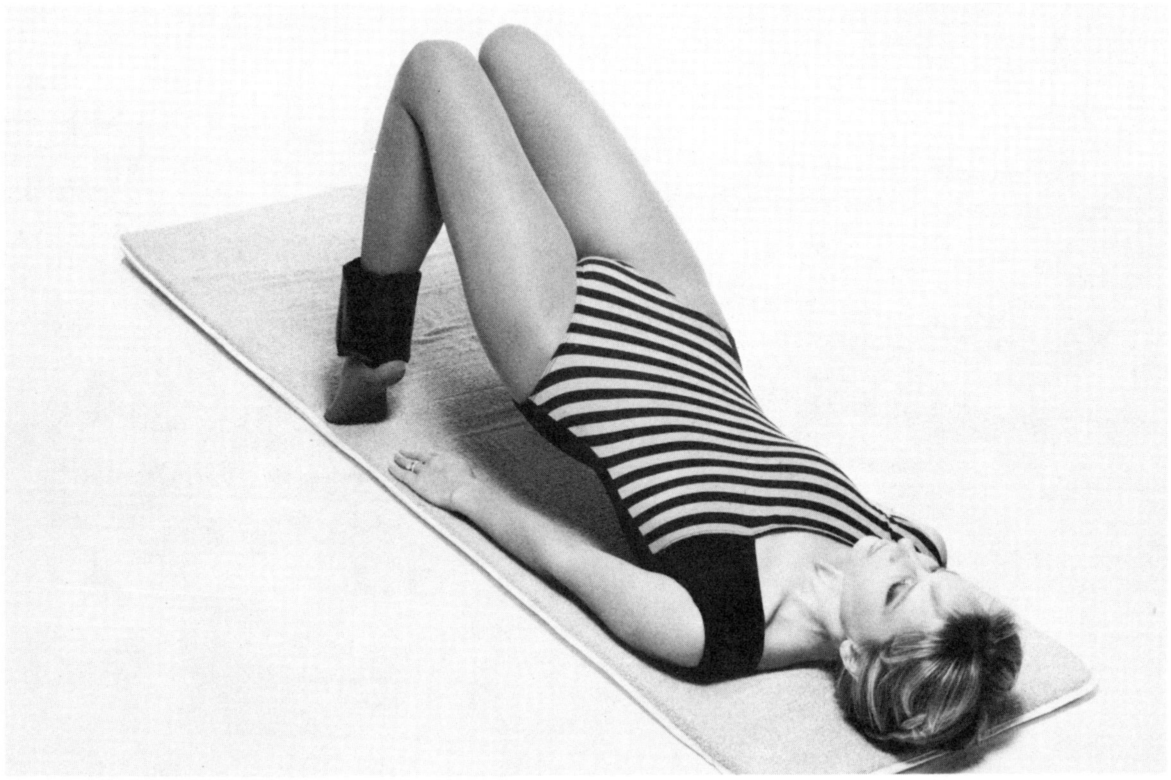

18. Spider: In same position, with weight on shoulders and feet, lift your heels off the mat. Bring one leg toward chest, knee bent. Then extend leg, hold, and return to original position.

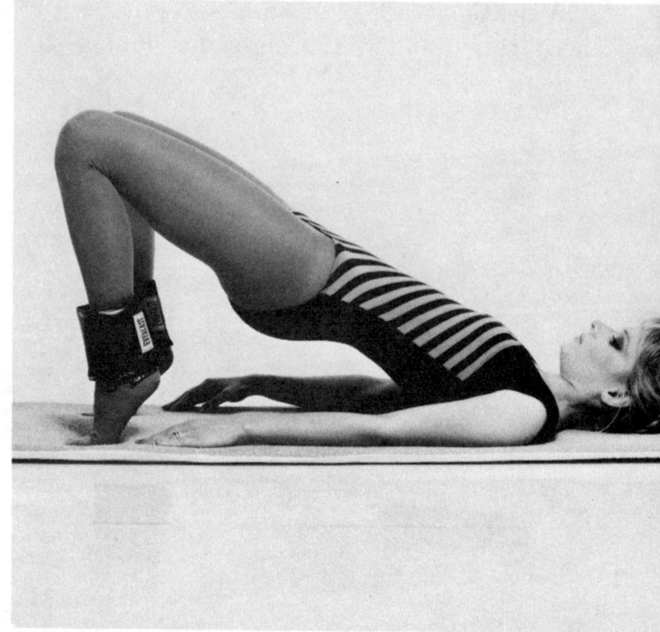

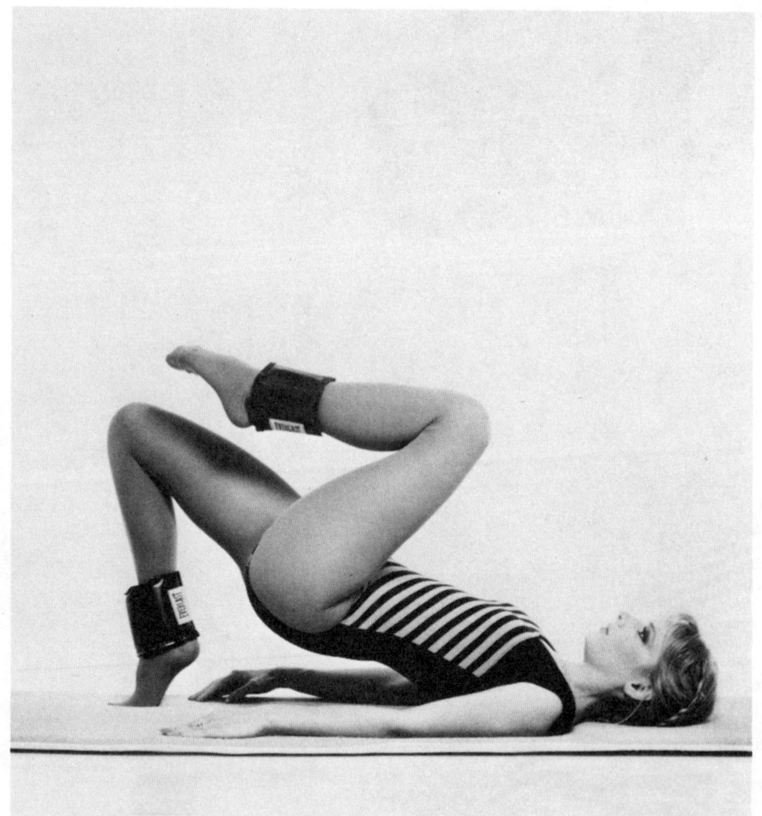

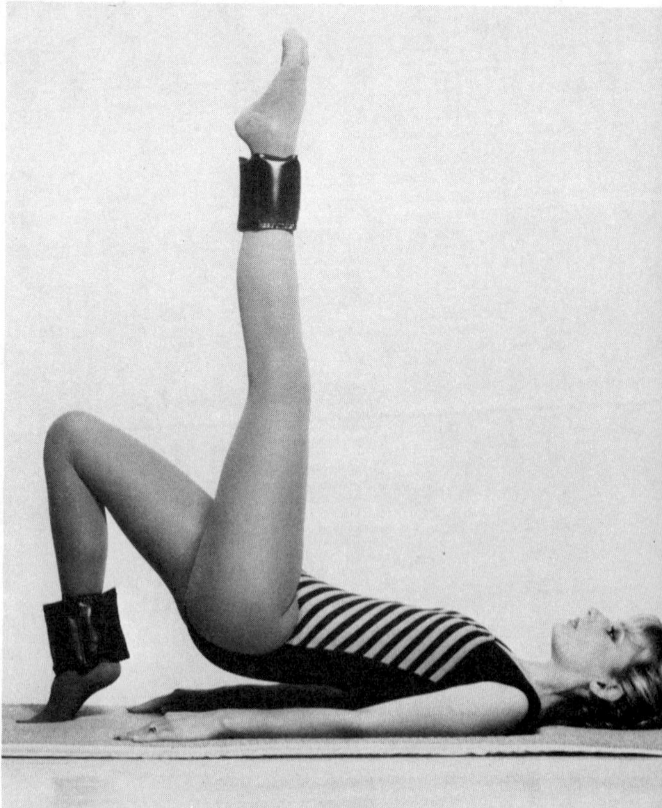

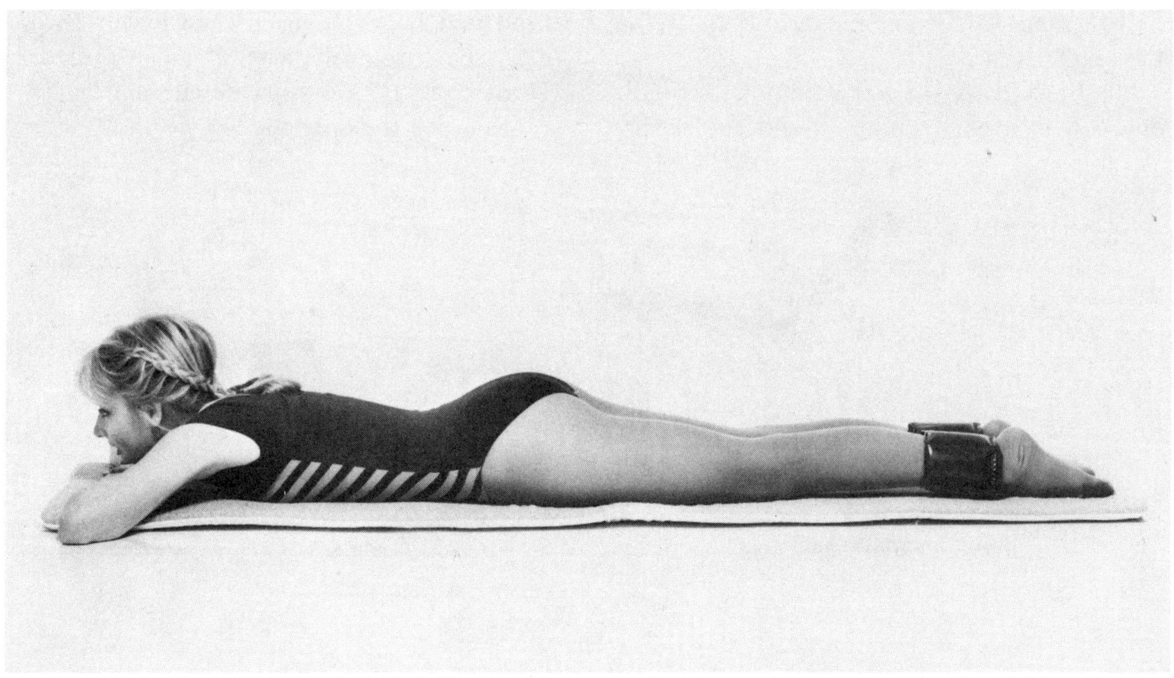

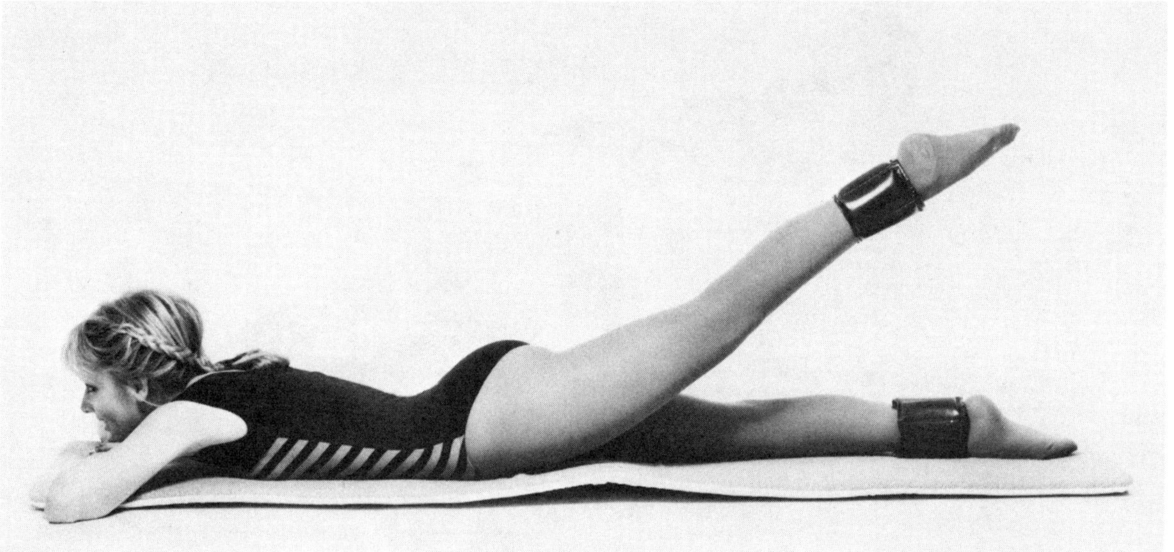

Great! Now roll over onto your stomach and do:

19. Back Lifts: Tighten seat (both sides) and lift one leg about a foot off the floor, keeping toes pointed. Lower and repeat, no more than 20 times. Repeat with opposite leg.

Now, come up to your hands and knees (on the mat):

20. Back Leg Lifts: Looking straight ahead with back straight, extend one leg behind you to seat height, then lower. Do not allow back to arch; keep stomach pulled in. Do as many lifts as you can with one leg, then repeat with the opposite leg.

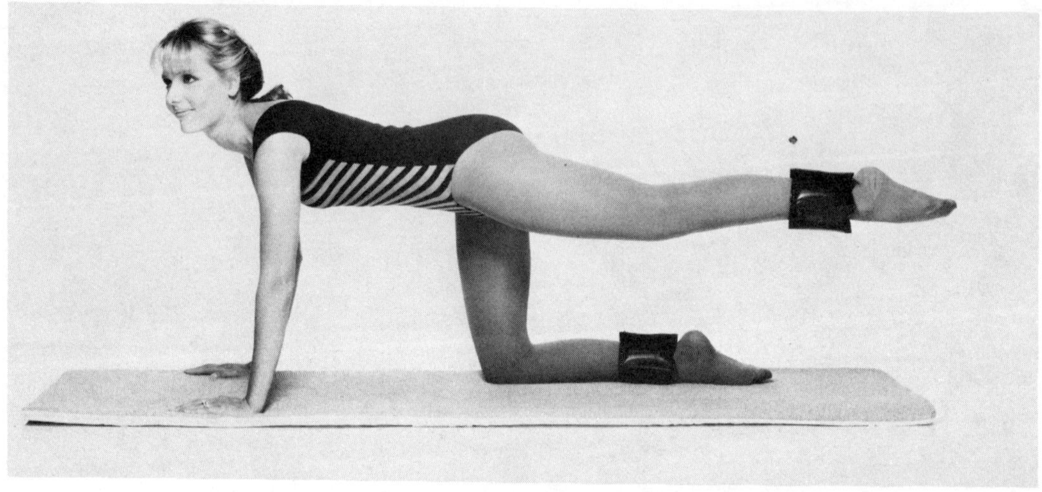

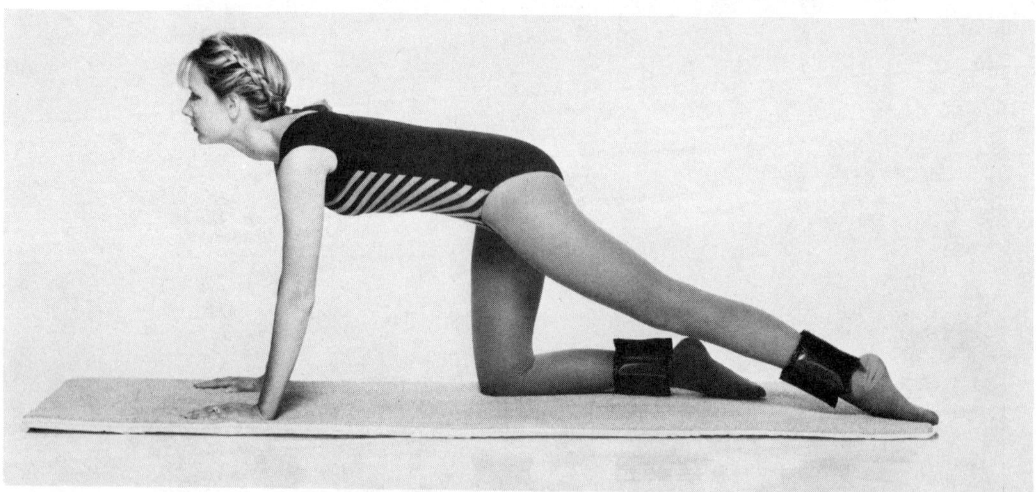

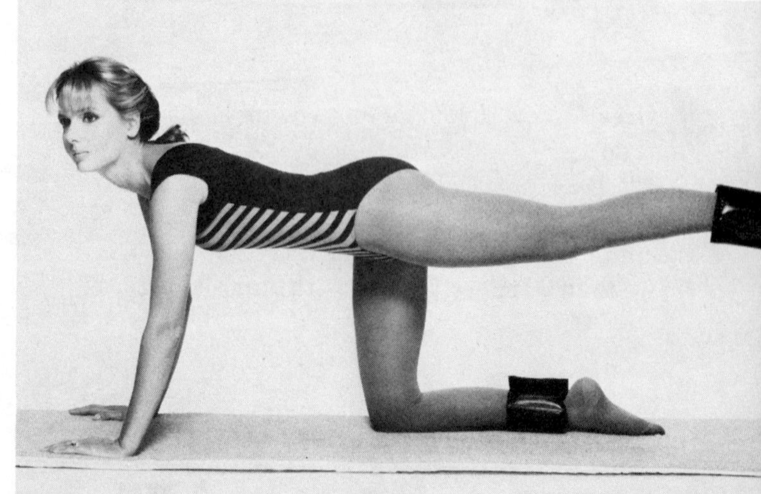

Variation: On alternate days, do as above, but with foot flexed.

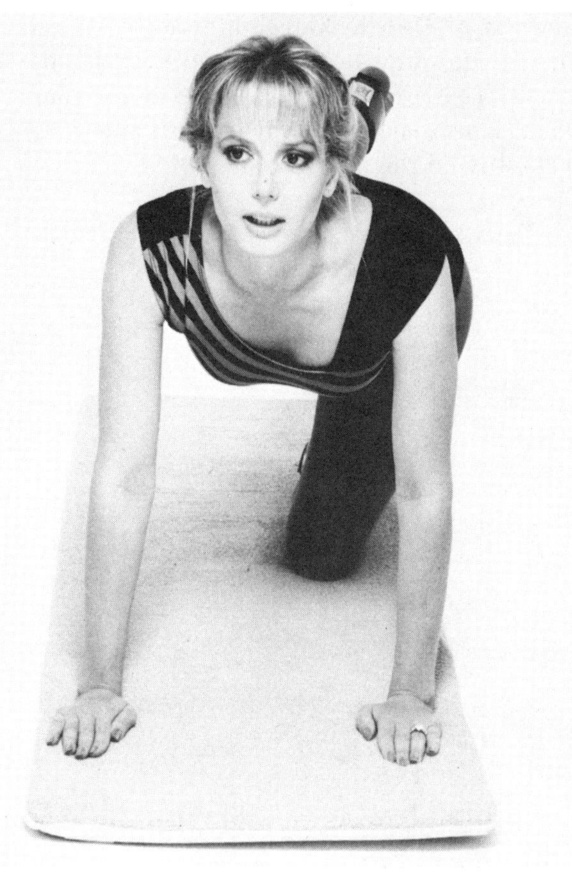

21. Butt Chopper: Still on hands and knees, tummy tucked in, seat tight, extend your right leg behind you. Swing it out to the right and touch the floor. Without pausing, swing it to the left, crossing over your left leg. Return to starting position and complete several repetitions; then switch legs.

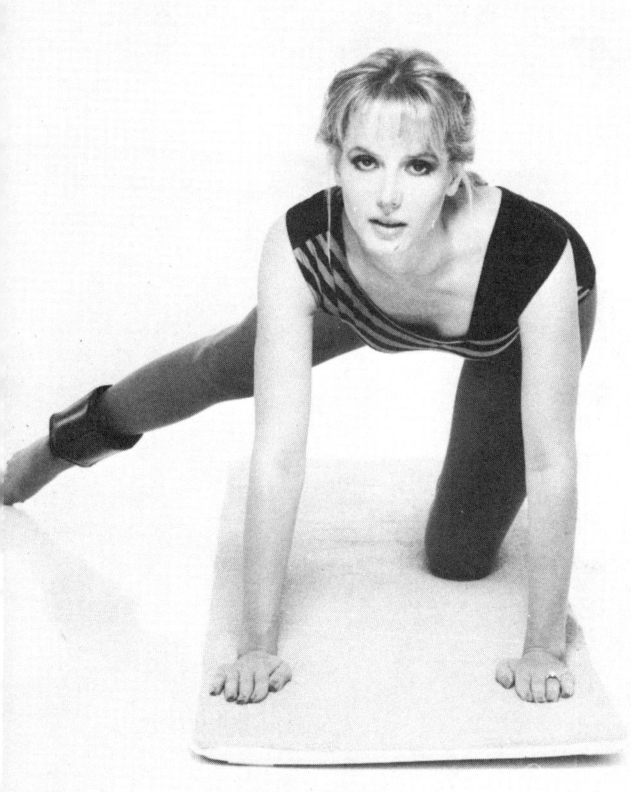

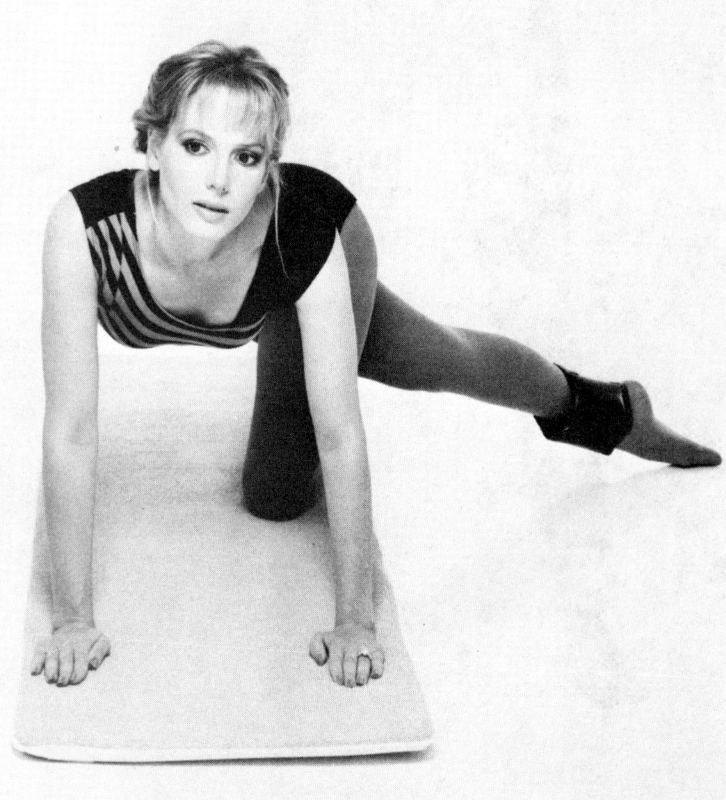

Now stand up. (Sure, you can.):

22. Plié: Stand with legs apart, seat tucked in and back straight. Lower your torso as far as you can while bending your knees in a plié; then straighten legs and return to standing position. Keep your hands out in front of you for balance, or on your waist. Knees should be turned out, and your heels stay on the floor throughout.

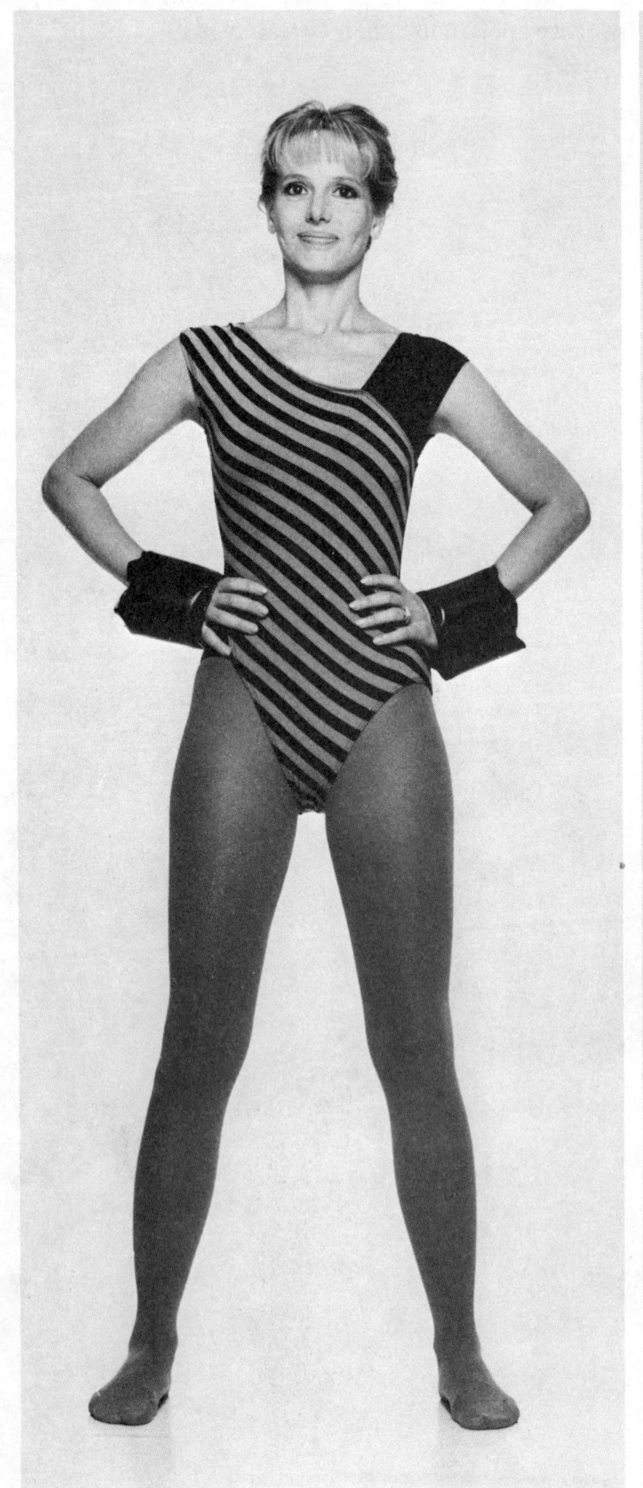

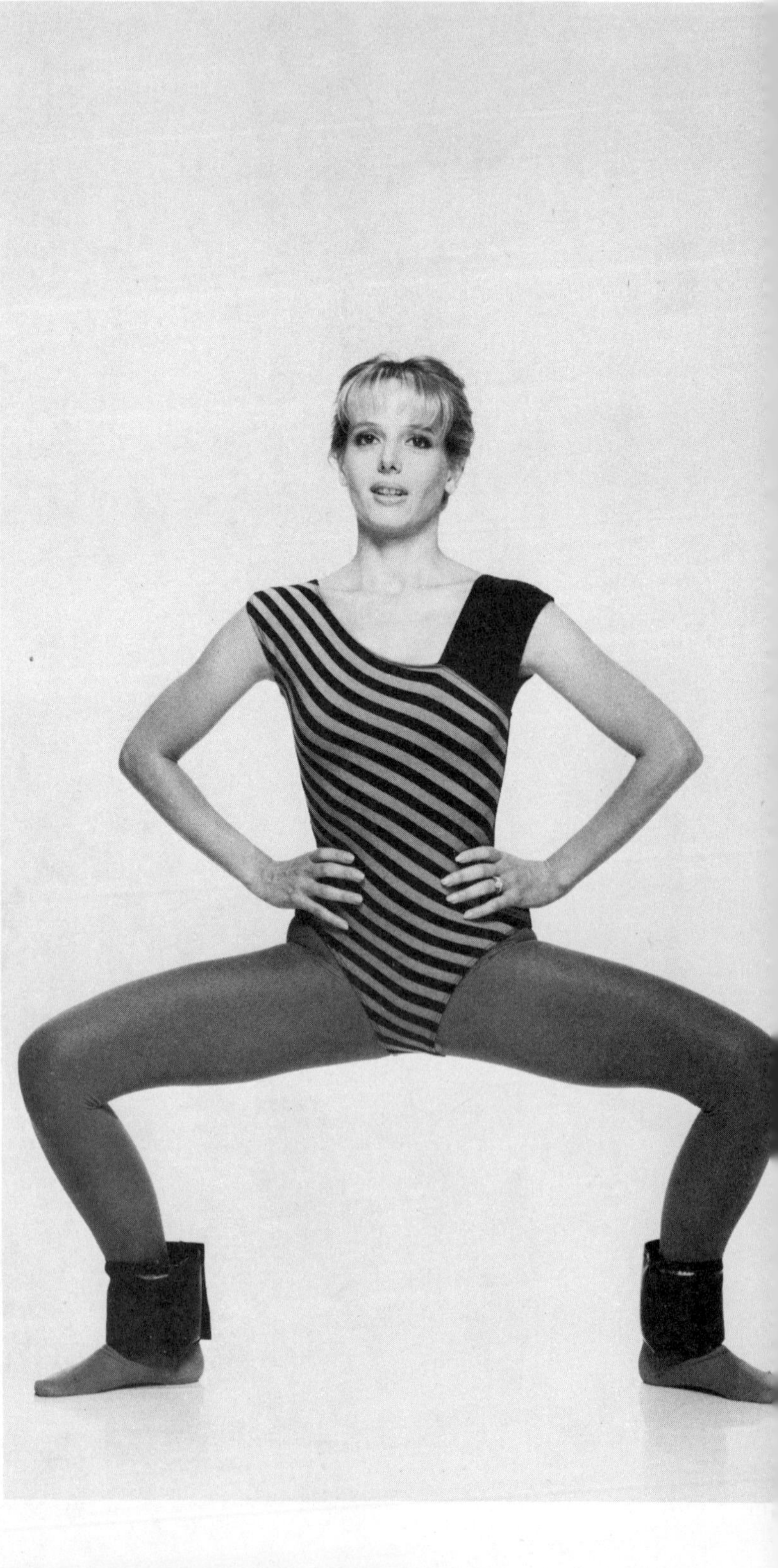

23. Plié with Heels Up: Repeat as above, but lift heels off the floor when you are in the plié. Again, lower as far as possible, keeping heels raised and seat tucked, then straighten legs.

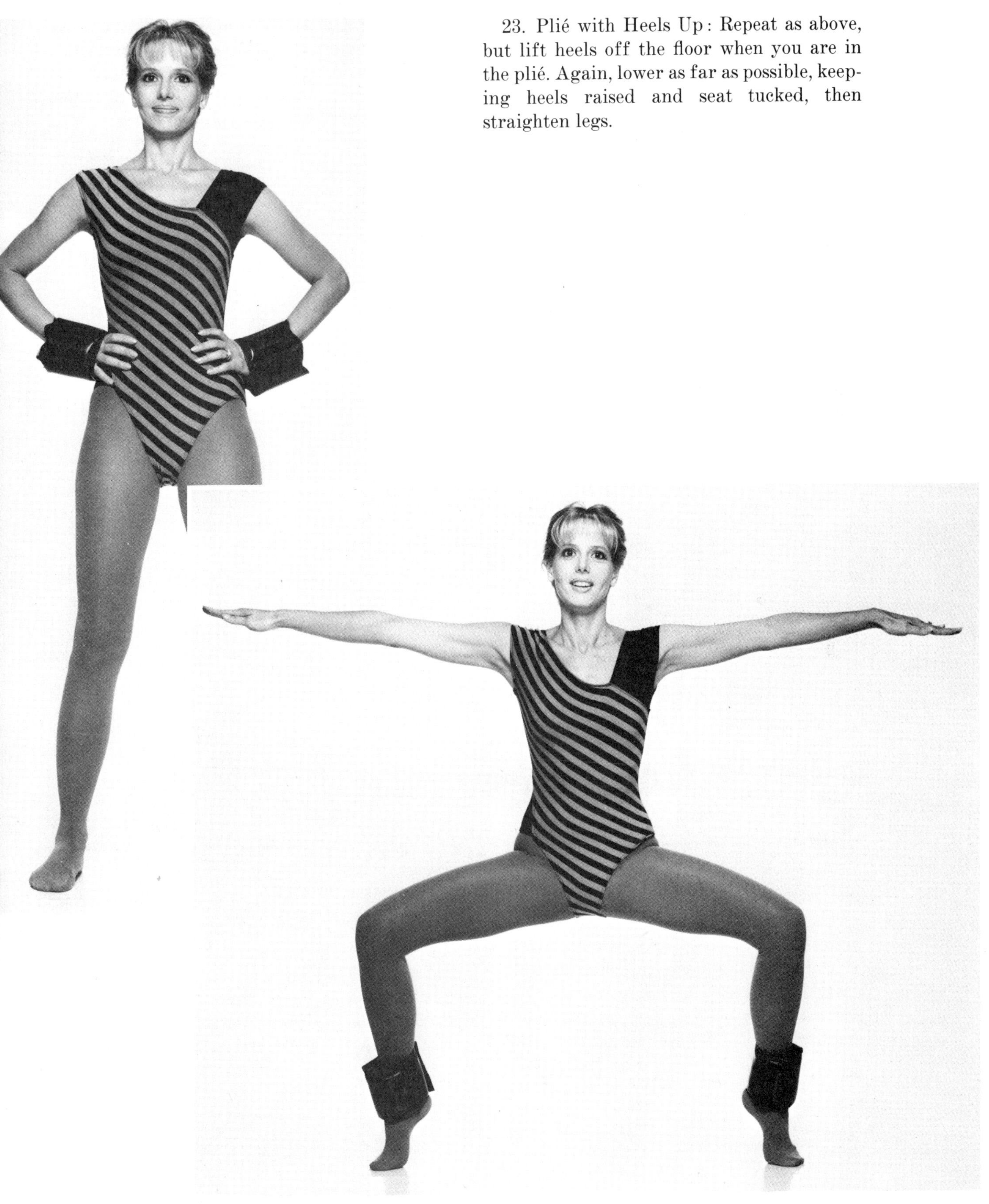

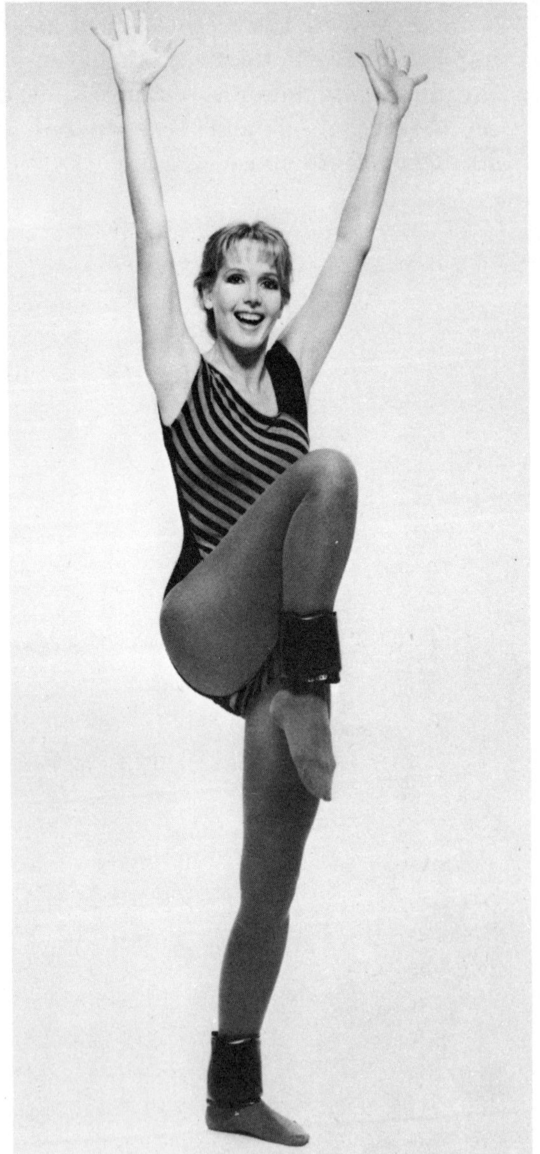

24. Leg Marching: Standing with tummy tucked and seat tight, raise and lower each leg in turn and march in place. Bring knees as high as possible, keeping toes pointed, arms raised. This is a good cool-down.

AVOIDING PAIN

It's not hard to strain your body when you are exercising, especially if you are careless. If you get too enthusiastic about a sport or exercise routine, you can be sore—or sorry—the next day. I've even ended up in bed for three days after a thrilling session in a class in New York. (What a class! I did everything like a pro! I felt wonderful! The next day I all but needed a wheelchair.) I have not, however, had any pain or injuries since using my own Work-Off—one of the reasons I like it. If you never go over your endurance limit, you will never be hurt. You do a *little* more each day without killing yourself. To avoid pain, with both my Work-Off and any other sport or exercise plan:

- Always warm up thoroughly.
- Exercise on a consistent basis. Weekend athletes have the most injuries.
- If you feel fatigued, quit.
- If you have pain, quit. Never exercise with pain without a doctor's permission.
- Remember, increasing weight and/or repetitions will build muscles, so do this only if that's what you want. Otherwise, maintain repetitions somewhere between 8 and 100, staying with 1-pound weights.
- Use an exercise mat. An uncovered floor is murder on your body—it's too hard. Jumping on an uncovered floor will cause shin splits.
- Cool down with stretching or a special technique at the end of each session.
- If you play sports on a regular basis or enjoy a particular class or go jogging, you are probably doing enough. Pick up exercises that work on your problem areas.
- If you feel you may have overdone, take a hot bath.

R.I.C.E. HELPS

If you do have an injury, R.I.C.E. helps:

*R*est: Too much movement can make an injury worse. If pain continues beyond twenty-four hours, get a doctor's opinion. He or she will guide you as to how much rest is best. (Too much rest is not good either.)

*I*ce: Apply ice (wrapped in a towel if you have no ice bag) to the injured area—this will curb swelling and numb nerves. Keep the ice pack on for about 15–30 minutes—no longer than a half-hour, because you can harm your skin.

*C*ompression: After the ice treatment, add an elastic bandage to keep swelling to a minimum. Just don't wrap up too tightly or you'll cut off the blood flow.

*E*levation: Keeping the injured part of your body elevated can help reduce swelling. Prop up your sorry limb on pillows, or use a chair as a resting place.

Always get medical advice after twenty-four hours of discomfort. (Sooner, if needed.) A telephone conversation may save you money—and pain. If you are a real jock, you may need a sports-medicine specialist; you can now find one in most big cities.

WHY EXERCISE WORKS

Exercise is invaluable for five reasons:

1. It keeps the body looking and working the way it should.
2. It helps you maintain your weight and tone the muscles.
3. It gives you confidence that comes from a feeling of strength.

4. Just moving about in your daily life becomes easier.

5. It releases tension and is therapeutic.

Marissa was driving her small foreign sports car through one of L.A.'s canyons. Coming around a curve at 40 mph, she saw a stalled car. To avoid hitting it, she banked her own auto. The car jumped the curb, rolled and pitched over a cliff. Marissa got out after the first roll and escaped with only scratches. In the emergency room to which she was rushed for tests, the doctors credited Marissa's lack of injury to her daily exercise routine. Because she was in prime condition, she was *able* to get out of that car. Someone who was not in good shape would have gone over the cliff.

Paulina also had a scare. She went to visit some friends who had a cabin near Jackson Hole, Wyoming. A city sophisticate, Paulina pictured herself sitting happily in front of a fireplace under an old-fashioned quilt drinking hot chocolate and reading a novel. Her friends picked her up at the airport and drove her in their Jeep to their snowbound cabin. It was a half-mile walk from the road to the cabin, in chest-high snow. Not being in good shape, unused to the altitude, Paulina suffered severe chest pains and had to be carried the last quarter-mile. She left the next day, vowing to get into shape before her condition cost her her life.

Julia shaped up for summer by dieting assiduously. Not one for sweating, she thought she could regulate her weight by controlling her food intake. What she didn't know is that 85 percent of the people who lose weight gain it back if they do not accompany their weight-loss plan with an exercise program.

IT'S ALL YOURS

If you eat well-balanced meals and get the right combination of exercise, your body will shape up and take on the dimensions you have dreamed of. With discipline, you can make your body do many wonderful things. (You may never get taller or shorter, but almost everything else is in your control.) More important, you will set a pattern for the rest of your life that will make good health and beauty part of your lifestyle. No one can predict what the future will bring, but I *know* you'll handle whatever comes your way better because you've taken the time now to establish your identity and your personal best. It's all yours now.